CONTAGION OF VIOLENCE

Workshop Summary

Deepali M. Patel, Melissa A. Simon,
and Rachel M. Taylor, *Rapporteurs*

Forum on Global Violence Prevention
Board on Global Health

INSTITUTE OF MEDICINE *AND*
NATIONAL RESEARCH COUNCIL
OF THE NATIONAL ACADEMIES

THE NATIONAL ACADEMIES PRESS
Washington, D.C.
www.nap.edu

THE NATIONAL ACADEMIES PRESS   500 Fifth Street, NW   Washington, DC 20001

NOTICE: The project that is the subject of this report was approved by the Governing Board of the National Research Council, whose members are drawn from the councils of the National Academy of Sciences, the National Academy of Engineering, and the Institute of Medicine.

This study was supported by contracts between the National Academy of Sciences and the Department of Health and Human Services: Administration on Children, Youth and Families, Administration on Community Living, Office on Women's Health; Anheuser-Busch InBev; the Avon Foundation for Women; BD (Becton, Dickinson and Company); Catholic Health Initiatives; the Centers for Disease Control and Prevention; the Department of Education: Office of Safe and Healthy Students; the Department of Justice: National Institute of Justice; Eli Lilly and Company; the F. Felix Foundation; the Fetzer Institute; the Foundation to Promote Open Society; the Joyce Foundation; Kaiser Permanente; the National Institutes of Health: National Institute on Alcoholism and Alcohol Abuse, National Institute on Drug Abuse, Office of Research on Women's Health, John E. Fogarty International Center; the Robert Wood Johnson Foundation; and the Substance Abuse and Mental Health Services Administration. The views presented in this publication do not necessarily reflect the views of the organizations or agencies that provided support for the project.

International Standard Book Number-13: 978-0-309-26364-1
International Standard Book Number-10: 0-309-26364-6

Additional copies of this report are available from the National Academies Press, 500 Fifth Street, NW, Keck 360, Washington, DC 20001; (800) 624-6242 or (202) 334-3313; http://www.nap.edu.

For more information about the Institute of Medicine, visit the IOM home page at: www.iom.edu.

The serpent has been a symbol of long life, healing, and knowledge among almost all cultures and religions since the beginning of recorded history. The serpent adopted as a logotype by the Institute of Medicine is a relief carving from ancient Greece, now held by the Staatliche Museen in Berlin.

Suggested citation: IOM (Institute of Medicine) and NRC (National Research Council). 2013. *Contagion of violence: Workshop summary.* Washington, DC: The National Academies Press.

THE NATIONAL ACADEMIES
Advisers to the Nation on Science, Engineering, and Medicine

The **National Academy of Sciences** is a private, nonprofit, self-perpetuating society of distinguished scholars engaged in scientific and engineering research, dedicated to the furtherance of science and technology and to their use for the general welfare. Upon the authority of the charter granted to it by the Congress in 1863, the Academy has a mandate that requires it to advise the federal government on scientific and technical matters. Dr. Ralph J. Cicerone is president of the National Academy of Sciences.

The **National Academy of Engineering** was established in 1964, under the charter of the National Academy of Sciences, as a parallel organization of outstanding engineers. It is autonomous in its administration and in the selection of its members, sharing with the National Academy of Sciences the responsibility for advising the federal government. The National Academy of Engineering also sponsors engineering programs aimed at meeting national needs, encourages education and research, and recognizes the superior achievements of engineers. Dr. Charles M. Vest is president of the National Academy of Engineering.

The **Institute of Medicine** was established in 1970 by the National Academy of Sciences to secure the services of eminent members of appropriate professions in the examination of policy matters pertaining to the health of the public. The Institute acts under the responsibility given to the National Academy of Sciences by its congressional charter to be an adviser to the federal government and, upon its own initiative, to identify issues of medical care, research, and education. Dr. Harvey V. Fineberg is president of the Institute of Medicine.

The **National Research Council** was organized by the National Academy of Sciences in 1916 to associate the broad community of science and technology with the Academy's purposes of furthering knowledge and advising the federal government. Functioning in accordance with general policies determined by the Academy, the Council has become the principal operating agency of both the National Academy of Sciences and the National Academy of Engineering in providing services to the government, the public, and the scientific and engineering communities. The Council is administered jointly by both Academies and the Institute of Medicine. Dr. Ralph J. Cicerone and Dr. Charles M. Vest are chair and vice chair, respectively, of the National Research Council.

www.national-academies.org

PLANNING COMMITTEE FOR WORKSHOP ON THE CONTAGION OF VIOLENCE[1]

L. ROWELL HUESMANN (*Chair*), Amos N. Tversky Collegiate Professor of Psychology and Communication Studies; Director, Research Center for Group Dynamics, Institute for Social Research, The University of Michigan

JACQUELYN C. CAMPBELL, Anna D. Wolf Chair and Professor, Johns Hopkins University School of Nursing

BRIAN W. FLYNN, Adjunct Professor, Department of Psychiatry, Uniformed Services University of the Health Sciences; Associate Director, Center for the Study of Traumatic Stress, Uniformed Services University School of Medicine

GARY SLUTKIN, Executive Director, Cure Violence (formerly CeaseFire); Professor of Epidemiology and International Health, University of Illinois at Chicago School of Public Health

EVELYN TOMASZEWSKI, Senior Policy Advisor, Human Rights and International Affairs, National Association of Social Workers

CHARLOTTE WATTS, Professor in Social and Mathematical Epidemiology; Founding Director, Gender Violence and Health Centre, London School of Hygiene and Tropical Medicine

---

[1] Institute of Medicine planning committees are solely responsible for organizing the workshop, identifying topics, and choosing speakers. The responsibility for the published workshop summary rests with the workshop rapporteurs and the institution.

FORUM ON GLOBAL VIOLENCE PREVENTION[1]

JACQUELYN C. CAMPBELL (*Co-Chair*), Anna D. Wolf Chair and Professor, Johns Hopkins University School of Nursing

MARK L. ROSENBERG (*Co-Chair*), President and Chief Executive Officer, The Task Force for Global Health

ALBERT J. ALLEN, Senior Medical Fellow, Bioethics and Pediatric Capabilities, Global Medical Affairs and Development Center of Excellence, Eli Lilly and Company

CLARE ANDERSON, Deputy Commissioner, Administration on Children, Youth and Families, Department of Health and Human Services

FRANCES ASHE-GOINS, Deputy Director, Office on Women's Health, Department of Health and Human Services

KATRINA BAUM, Senior Research Officer, Office of Research Partnerships, National Institute of Justice, Department of Justice

SUSAN BISSELL, Associate Director, Child Protection Section, United Nations Children's Fund

ARTURO CERVANTES TREJO, General Director of Health Promotion for Mexico, Federal Ministry of Health, Mexico

XINQI DONG, Associate Director, Rush Institute for Healthy Aging; Associate Professor of Medicine, Behavioral Sciences, and Gerontological Nursing, Rush University Medical Center

AMIE GIANINO, Senior Global Director, Beer & Better World, Anheuser-Busch InBev

KATHY GREENLEE, Administrator, Administration on Community Living; Assistant Secretary for Aging, Administration on Aging, Department of Health and Human Services

RODRIGO V. GUERRERO, Mayor, Cali, Colombia

JOHN HAYES, Executive Director, National Network of Depression Centers

DAVID HEMENWAY, Director, Injury Control Research Center and the Youth Violence Prevention Center, Harvard University School of Public Health

FRANCES HENRY, Advisor, F. Felix Foundation

LARKE NAHME HUANG, Senior Advisor, Office of the Administrator, Substance Abuse and Mental Health Services Administration, Department of Health and Human Services

---

[1] Institute of Medicine Forums and Roundtables do not issue, review, or approve individual documents. The responsibility for the published workshop summary rests with the workshop rapporteurs and the institution.

L. ROWELL HUESMANN, Amos N. Tversky Collegiate Professor of Psychology and Communication Studies; Director, Research Center for Group Dynamics, Institute for Social Research, The University of Michigan

PAUL KESNER, Director, Safe and Supportive Schools Program, Office of Safe and Healthy Students, Department of Education

CAROL M. KURZIG, President, Avon Foundation for Women

JACQUELINE LLOYD, Health Scientist Administrator, Prevention Research Branch, Division of Epidemiology, Services and Prevention Research, National Institute on Drug Abuse

BRIGID McCAW, Medical Director, NCal Family Violence Prevention Program, Kaiser Permanente

JAMES A. MERCY, Special Advisor for Strategic Directions, Division of Violence Prevention, National Center for Injury Prevention and Control, Centers for Disease Control and Prevention

MARGARET M. MURRAY, Director, Global Alcohol Research Program, National Institute for Alcohol Abuse and Alcoholism, National Institutes of Health

MICHAEL PHILLIPS, Director, Suicide Research and Prevention Center, Shanghai Jiao Tong University School of Medicine

COLLEEN SCANLON, Senior Vice President, Advocacy, Catholic Health Initiatives

KRISTIN SCHUBERT, Interim Team Director, Public Health and Program Officer, Vulnerable Populations, Robert Wood Johnson Foundation

EVELYN TOMASZEWSKI, Senior Policy Advisor, Human Rights and International Affairs, National Association of Social Workers

ELIZABETH WARD, Chair, Violence Prevention Alliance, University of the West Indies, Mona Campus

IOM Staff

DEEPALI M. PATEL, Program Officer
RACHEL M. TAYLOR, Research Associate
MEGAN M. PEREZ, Senior Program Assistant
KATHERINE M. BLAKESLEE, Global Program Advisor
ALICIA DAVIS, Intern
MELISSA A. SIMON, Institute of Medicine Anniversary Fellow
JULIE WILTSHIRE, Financial Officer
PATRICK W. KELLEY, Director, Board on Global Health

Reviewers

This workshop summary has been reviewed in draft form by individuals chosen for their diverse perspectives and technical expertise, in accordance with procedures approved by the National Research Council's Report Review Committee. The purpose of this independent review is to provide candid and critical comments that will assist the institution in making its published workshop summary as sound as possible and to ensure that the workshop summary meets institutional standards for objectivity, evidence, and responsiveness to the study charge. The review comments and draft manuscript remain confidential to protect the integrity of the process. We wish to thank the following individuals for their review of this workshop summary:

DAVID ADDISS, Director, Children Without Worms, The Task Force for Global Health

BRIAN W. FLYNN, Adjunct Professor, Department of Psychiatry, Uniformed Services University of the Health Sciences; Associate Director, Center for the Study of Traumatic Stress, Uniformed Services University School of Medicine

VALERIE MAHOLMES, Director, Child and Family Processes/Child Maltreatment & Violence Program, *Eunice Kennedy Shriver* National Institute of Child Health and Human Development, National Institutes of Health

ZOE MENTEL, Policy Analyst, U.S. Department of Justice

EVELYN TOMASZEWSKI, Senior Policy Advisor, Human Rights and International Affairs, National Association of Social Workers

Although the reviewers listed above have provided many constructive comments and suggestions, they did not see the final draft of the workshop summary before its release. The review of this workshop summary was overseen by **Dyanne D. Affonso,** Director, Research Infrastructure, Office of Vice President of Research, University of Hawaii System. Appointed by the Institute of Medicine, she was responsible for making certain that an independent examination of this workshop summary was carried out in accordance with institutional procedures and that all review comments were carefully considered. Responsibility for the final content of this workshop summary rests entirely with the authors and the institution.

Acknowledgments

The Forum on Global Violence Prevention was established to develop multisectoral collaboration among stakeholders. Violence prevention is a crossdisciplinary field that could benefit from increased dialogue among researchers, policy makers, funders, and practitioners. As awareness of the insidious and pervasive nature of violence grows, so too does the imperative to mitigate and prevent it. The Forum seeks to illuminate and explore evidence-based approaches to the prevention of violence.

A number of individuals contributed to the development of this workshop and summary. These include a number of staff members from the Institute of Medicine and the National Academies: Pamela Bertelson, Daniel Bethea, Leigh Carroll, Marton Cavani, Angela Christian, Alicia Davis, Laura Harbold DeStefano, Pablo Flores, Meg Ginivan, Sandra Jones, Wendy Keenan, Patrick Kelley, Eileen Milner, Jose Portillo, Patsy Powell, Samantha Robotham, Julie Wiltshire, and Sarah Ziegenhorn. The Forum staff, including Deepali Patel, Megan Perez, and Rachel Taylor, also put forth considerable effort to ensure this workshop's success.

The planning committee contributed several hours of service to develop and execute the agenda, with the guidance of Forum membership. Reviewers also provided thoughtful remarks in reading the draft manuscript. Finally, these efforts would not be possible without the work of the Forum membership itself, an esteemed body of individuals dedicated to the concept that violence is preventable.

The overall successful functioning of the Forum and its activities depends on the generosity of its sponsors. Financial support for the Forum on

Global Violence Prevention is provided by the Department of Health and Human Services: Administration on Children, Youth and Families, Administration on Community Living, Office on Women's Health; Anheuser-Busch InBev; the Avon Foundation for Women; BD (Becton, Dickinson and Company); Catholic Health Initiatives; the Centers for Disease Control and Prevention; the Department of Education: Office of Safe and Healthy Students; the Department of Justice: National Institute of Justice; Eli Lilly and Company; the F. Felix Foundation; the Fetzer Foundation; the Foundation to Promote Open Society; the Joyce Foundation; Kaiser Permanente; the National Institutes of Health: National Institute on Alcoholism and Alcohol Abuse, National Institute on Drug Abuse, Office of Research on Women's Health, John E. Fogarty International Center; the Robert Wood Johnson Foundation; and the Substance Abuse and Mental Health Services Administration.

Contents

xiii

APPENDIXES

1

Introduction[1]

The past 25 years have seen a major paradigm shift in the field of violence prevention, from the assumption that violence is inevitable to the recognition that violence is preventable. Part of this shift has occurred in thinking about why violence occurs, and where intervention points might lie. In exploring the occurrence of violence, researchers have recognized the tendency for violent acts to cluster, to spread from place to place, and to mutate from one type to another. Furthermore, violent acts are often preceded or followed by other violent acts. Contextual and social factors play a role in increasing or reducing the risk of violence; such factors might exist at community or individual levels.

In the field of public health, such a process has also been seen in the infectious disease model, in which an agent or vector initiates a specific biological pathway leading to symptoms of disease and infectivity. The agent transmits from individual to individual, and levels of the disease in the population above the expected rate constitute an epidemic. Although violence does not have a readily observable biological agent as an initiator, it can follow similar epidemiological pathways. Just as with those infected by microbial agents, those exposed to violence have varying levels of resilience

---

[1] The planning committee's role was limited to planning the workshop. The workshop summary was prepared by the workshop rapporteurs as a factual summary of what occurred at the workshop. Statements, recommendations, and opinions expressed are those of individual presenters and participants and are not necessarily endorsed or verified by the Forum, the Institute of Medicine, or the National Research Council, and they should not be construed as reflecting any group consensus.

and susceptibility. In addition, the influence of the environment can play a major role not only in symptomology, but also in transmission.

On April 30-May 1, 2012, the Institute of Medicine (IOM) Forum on Global Violence Prevention convened a workshop to explore the contagious nature of violence (see Box 1-1 for the Statement of Task). Part of the Forum's mandate is to engage in multisectoral, multidirectional dialogue that explores crosscutting, evidence-based approaches to violence prevention, and the Forum has convened four workshops to this point exploring various elements of violence prevention. The workshops are designed to examine such approaches from multiple perspectives and at multiple levels of society. In particular, the workshop on the contagion of violence focused on exploring the epidemiology of the contagion, describing possible processes and mechanisms by which violence is transmitted, examining how contextual factors mitigate or exacerbate the issue, and illuminating ways in which the contagion of violence might be interrupted. Speakers were invited to share the progress and outcomes of their work and to engage in a dialogue exploring the gaps and opportunities in the field. It should be noted that, while the infectious disease model was utilized as a framework for common language, not all speakers approached the issue of contagion literally. These differing approaches allowed for an emerging exploration of this issue, and one that might benefit from future exploration and research.

BOX 1-1
Statement of Task

The contagion of violence is a universal phenomenon, occurring at all levels of society and affecting a broad spectrum of individuals. It occurs globally, within all societies, and is transmitted through interpersonal relationships, families, peer groups, neighborhoods, and cultures. The Institute of Medicine will convene a 2-day workshop to explore the contagion of violence and how it can be prevented and eventually ended. The workshop will emphasize the challenge in low- and middle-income countries, where the burden of violence is the greatest.

The public workshop will be organized and conducted by an ad hoc committee to examine (1) the contagious nature of violence, (2) the relationship between the contagion of violence and epidemics of violence, and (3) how contagions of violence can be prevented or ended.

The committee will develop the workshop agenda, select and invite speakers and discussants, and moderate the discussions. Experts will be drawn from the public and private sectors as well as from academic organizations to allow for multilateral, evidence-based discussions. Following the conclusion of the workshop, an individually authored summary of the event will be prepared by a designated rapporteur.

The World Health Organization (WHO) defines violence as "the intentional use of physical force or power, threatened or actual, against oneself, another person, or against a group or community that either results in or has a high likelihood of resulting in injury, death, psychological harm, maldevelopment, or deprivation" (WHO, 2002). WHO further categorizes violence into seven types: child abuse, elder abuse, sexual violence, intimate partner violence, youth violence, collective violence, and self-directed violence.

The workshop was planned by a formally appointed committee of the IOM, whose members created an agenda and identified relevant speakers. Because the topic is large and the field is broad, presentations at this event represent only a sample of the research currently being undertaken. Speakers were chosen to present a global, balanced perspective, but by no means a comprehensive one. Working within the limitations imposed by its time and resource constraints, the planning committee members chose speakers who could provide diverse perspectives on which further discussion could occur. The agenda for this workshop can be found in Appendix A. The speakers' presentations and the audio recordings of the workshop can also be found on the website for the workshop: http://iom.edu/contagionofviolence.

ORGANIZATION OF THE REPORT

This summary provides an account of the presentations given at the workshop. Opinions expressed within this summary are not those of the IOM, the National Research Council, the Forum on Global Violence Prevention, or their agents, but rather of the presenters themselves. Such statements are the views of the speakers and do not reflect conclusions or recommendations of a formally appointed committee. This summary was authored by designated rapporteurs based on the workshop presentations and discussions and does not represent the views of the institution, nor does it constitute a full or exhaustive overview of the field.

The workshop summary covers the major topics that arose during the 2-day workshop. It is organized by important elements of the infectious disease model so as to present the contagion of violence in a larger context and in a more compelling and comprehensive way. The topics and key points presented in this summary were the most frequent, crosscutting, and essential elements that arose from the various presentations of the workshop, but the choice of these topics does not represent the views of the IOM or a formal consensus process.

The first part of this report consists of four chapters that provide a summary of the workshop: Patterns of Transmission of Violence (Chapter 2), Processes and Mechanisms of the Contagion of Violence (Chapter 3), The Role of Contextual Factors in the Contagion of Violence (Chapter 4), and Contagion and Interruption in Practice (Chapter 5). The second part consists of submitted papers and commentary from speakers regarding the substance of the work they presented at the workshop. These papers were solicited from speakers in order to offer further information about their work and this field; not all speakers contributed papers. Finally, the appendixes contain the workshop agenda (Appendix A), a glossary (Appendix B), and the speakers' biographies (Appendix C).

REFERENCE

WHO (World Health Organization). 2002. *World report on violence and health*. Geneva, Switzerland: WHO.

Part I

Workshop Summary

2

Patterns of Transmission of Violence

While it is commonly accepted knowledge that violence begets violence, many workshop speakers emphasized that epidemiological research methods can reveal the ways in which violence spreads, both from one act of violence to many and as a spillover from one type of violence to others. Institute of Medicine (IOM) Board on Global Health Director Patrick Kelley noted that in epidemiology, when trying to understand an infectious disease, the methodology begins with a description of the distribution of cases in person, place, and time. Therefore, an epidemiological survey of the contagion of violence should begin with what different types of violence exist, who is infected, and where and when the violence spreads.

Such a methodology is not new to violence research and prevention. Speaker Valerie Maholmes from the *Eunice Kennedy Shriver* National Institute of Child Health & Human Development (NICHD) pointed out that, in 1993, a National Institutes of Health panel recommended that research funding priorities in the area of violence should place an emphasis on the context in which violence occurs, and, 10 years later, NICHD led an initiative calling for research on the epidemiology of children exposed to violence. The data presented by many of the workshop speakers highlighted the epidemiological approaches that have been applied to research on and interventions to prevent multiple types of violence.

TYPES OF TRANSMISSION AND SYNDROMES

Speaker and planning committee member Gary Slutkin of the University of Illinois at Chicago defined infectious disease transmission as occurring when an individual or population is exposed to the particular disease and has an increased likelihood of developing the disease. An individual who is inflicted with a disease exhibits some form of symptoms, which vary depending on the disease. Dr. Slutkin suggested that a symptom of violence can be physically injuring another person; speaker Madelyn Gould of Columbia University added that self-directed injury also can be a symptom of violence. Many workshop speakers noted that violence can be transmitted through either direct victimization or merely through witnessing violence.

The incubation period from when the exposure occurs and until disease symptoms develop can vary. As Forum co-chair Mark Rosenberg of the Task Force for Global Health stated, "it can be a long time between something first affecting a person and when it shows up, so [for example] within a family, children [who are] exposed at a very young age may have its impact much later." To highlight the similarity between varying incubation periods of violence and other infectious diseases, Dr. Slutkin made a comparison between a young child's exposure to tuberculosis and child abuse. In cases of tuberculosis, reactivation of the disease can occur when the child is in his or her teens or twenties, just as someone exposed to child abuse may become a perpetrator of dating violence or intimate partner violence during adolescence or later in life.

Several workshop speakers pointed to research showing that violence manifests and spreads as different syndromes—collective, interpersonal, and self-directed—and transmission can result in an infection of the same type of violence to which an individual was exposed or as a different syndrome.

Transmission Within Types of Violence

Dr. Slutkin cited evidence that exposure to community violence can lead to perpetration of community violence (Kelly, 2010). The 2011 London riots are an example of how community violence can quickly spread. Furthermore, large-scale political violence can spread to additional perpetration of political violence, as were the cases in World War II and the mass killings in Rwanda in the 1990s, which Dr. Slutkin cited as examples.

Like the spread of acts of collective violence, evidence shows that exposure to interpersonal violence leads to additional acts of interpersonal violence. Speaker and planning committee member Charlotte Watts of the London School of Hygiene and Tropical Medicine noted that there is evidence of the relationship between intimate partner violence and other types of interpersonal violence. She cited the relationship between early exposures to child sexual abuse, violent households, and harsh punishment as a child, and a woman being more vulnerable later in life to experiencing violence (Abramsky et al., 2011). Furthermore, she pointed to evidence that similar early exposure to violence for men is linked to increased likelihood of perpetrating violence. This early exposure to violence can be the child being directly violated or witnessing violence in the home. Additionally, childhood exposure to interpersonal violence in the home can lead to the child's perpetration of interpersonal violence against peers later in life, through bullying and dating violence (Crooks, 2011).

The contagion of self-directed violence also has been shown to exist; Dr. Gould noted that the evidence base on the impact of media reporting on suicide, suicide clusters, and adolescent exposure to a suicidal peer has shown an increase in cases of suicidal behavior, both directly and indirectly (Gould, 1990).

Transmission Among Types of Violence

Violence spreads not only as one act of violence to many, but as one act of violence to acts of other types of violence. Many speakers cited evidence of this spread between types of violence. Dr. Watts noted that there is evidence that suicidal behavior can manifest from exposure to other forms of violence; women's experience with intimate partner violence is linked to increased suicidality (Devries et al., 2011). Similarly, exposure to collective violence can lead to increased rates of intimate partner violence and other forms of interpersonal violence. Speaker Eric Dubow of Bowling Green State University presented evidence that links exposure to ethnopolitical violence and multiple forms of interpersonal violence. He cited studies that support ethnopolitical violence as a higher level stressor that increases other forms of violence at other ecological levels, such as violence within the community, within the schools, and within the family (Dubow et al., 2010; Cummings et al., 2010, 2011). In addition to spread through ethnopolitical violence, exposure to community violence also can lead to an increase in family violence (Mullins et al., 2004).

Dr. Slutkin commented that the manifestation of family violence resulting from exposure to ethnopolitical violence is particularly interesting for the disease model because there is no rational explanation why exposure to violence from an enemy would lead to perpetration against family members. He suggested that this type of transmission shows that violence spreads not for logical reasons, but because it is a communicable disease. He compared the manifestation of different syndromes of violence to the emergence of different syndromes in other diseases, such as bubonic versus pneumonic plague.

Understanding the relationship between multiple forms of violence is important for detecting risk factors for the manifestation of future transmissions of violence, and the contagion model can be used to illuminate such pathways. Dr. Gould provided an example that highlighted the importance of such research, including a study that examined multiple forms of violence. Such research, rather than that which is singularly focused on one type of violence, can avoid missing unexpected links among the multiple forms of violence. For example, suicide clusters are primarily a male phenomenon; however, one exception has been among African American girls in gang-related situations where they have been coerced into gang membership and sexual behaviors. Their exposure to collective and interpersonal violence has led to an association with a contagion of suicide within the group.

SUSCEPTIBILITY AND CONTRIBUTING FACTORS

Dr. Slutkin noted that, like other infectious diseases, not everyone who is exposed to violence exhibits symptoms and many individuals can act as carriers without serving as a vector. Physical symptoms of violence are inflicted on those individuals who are susceptible to the disease. Many speakers discussed contributing factors that affect an individual's or a population's susceptibility to violence. Many of these factors apply to contagion within and across multiple types of violence.

Social Norms

Many workshop speakers commented that the contagion of violence is dependent on norms associated with violence. A disconnection from or erosion of positive social norms makes individuals and communities more susceptible to the contagion of violence. In citing an example of youth violence in New York City, speaker Jeffrey Fagan of Columbia Law School noted the disconnection between the social norms of the police and the youth as a contributing factor in the contagion of violence. He suggested that there is an extraordinary detachment of youth from the social norms that the police are trying to enforce, which creates a cynicism about the legal system. The higher levels of cynicism about the legal system lead to detachment from the moral and social norms of the law and result in higher rates of violence in those areas. Dr. Dubow noted that there is evidence that violence resulting from conflicts with out-groups is also generalized toward in-group members in society, showing a gradual, consistent, and continuous process of erosion of basic social norms regarding violence in society.

Many workshop speakers noted that although deteriorating social norms can increase susceptibility to violence, changing social norms can be a tool for interrupting the contagion. Dr. Gould noted that recent suicide preventive interventions are focusing on changing peer norms in schools. A program for high school students called Sources of Strength is focused on encouraging students to go to a trusted adult if the student is concerned a peer may be at risk for suicide. The program works by changing norms through emphasizing the importance of help-seeking behavior. Dr. Watts cited violence prevention intervention models and evaluations from Brazil and from South Africa that show that active engagement of men and boys to redefine masculinity can reduce the perpetration of intimate partner violence.

Network Density

Dr. Fagan noted that the contagion of violence is primarily a social network phenomenon, and increased network density increases the risk of violence transmission. He cited the social network density within public housing communities as an example of such a phenomenon. However, the increased risk is not a factor merely of the density, but the transmission of norms and cultural software that is amplified and reinforced through the network structure. Within insular social networks where violence and danger are learned norms, there is little opportunity to introduce a different kind of social norms model that could teach risk regulation behavior and reduce violence transmission. Dr. Fagan showed a map of incidents of gun-related violence in New York City. The mapping demonstrated the formation of co-offending networks that coalesce around individuals who originally had no or minimal connections, but over time became tighter and tighter social networks.

Dr. Gould also presented the evidence on suicidal behavior based on exposure to a suicide within a peer network. She noted that there has not been that much research in this area, but the majority of the 16 studies that have been done have found a significant association between being exposed to a suicidal peer and the subsequent suicide attempt with odds ratio from 2.8-11.0.

Dose-Response Effect

The dose-response effect, that is, the role of increased and repeated exposure to violence, was brought up by several speakers. Dr. Dubow commented that the more ethnopolitical violence to which children are exposed, the greater the occurrences of community, school, and family violence, and individual aggressive behavior. Dr. Gould cited that more than 50 studies on non-fictional stories of suicide reported in the media have consistently shown that there is a dose-response effect; the more coverage and the more dramatic the coverage, the greater the increase in suicide rates. The reverse also has been shown; suicide rates go down following a decrease in the number of media reports on suicide (Motto, 1970; Hagihara et al., 2007). Dr. Watts suggested there is a dose-response relationship in the contagion of intimate partner violence as well; if both the man and the woman come into the relation with histories of violence, the risk of violence occurring increases.

Media

Forum member and planning committee chair Rowell Huesmann of the University of Michigan stated that evidence has clearly shown that media violence promotes the contagion of violence significantly and substantially. Dr. Gould highlighted the role of the media on suicide clusters. She cited that the most consistent finding is related to the dose-response effect, which is that there are significant increases in suicides when the frequency of media reporting on suicides increases. In addition to increases based on the number of reports, there is a greater likelihood of an increase in suicide when the headlines of the stories are dramatic and when the coverage is on the front page. Dr. Gould pointed to evidence that interventions targeting media coverage have been shown to decrease suicide contagion. She cited an example of media guidelines in Vienna focused on suicides on the subway system in which there was a 75 percent decrease after the guideline implementation. Despite the role of media on transmissions of suicide, she cautioned that media reporting on suicide alone does not lead to suicide contagion; the host, audience, and observer's preexisting susceptibility all play a role as well.

Dr. Gould noted that while there is a body of evidence on the relationship between traditional media reporting and suicide contagion, the effects of the Internet have not been well studied. She suggested that trying to determine the effects of the Internet on suicide contagion is challenging because the speed at which the communication is shared is faster than anything seen before or even envisioned. Dr. Fagan suggested there is a paradox when it comes to the role of the media and community violence. From one perspective, the more time a youth spends on the Internet, the less time he or she is out in the community engaging in violent behavior. However, youth are exposed to violent content through the Internet. That raises many other questions about, for example, what the dose-response curves are and what personal characteristics are mediating factors. Dr. Watts also commented on the paradox of violence and the Internet. As an example, she stated that individuals who have leanings toward pedophilia may be in scattered physical locations, but the Internet provides an opportunity to link up with like-minded people and to reinforce and condone those behaviors and maybe lead to action. But she also acknowledged that the Internet has provided extensive opportunities in terms of promoting alternatives and providing youth different forms of relationships and ways to have relationships.

Youth Factors

Several workshop speakers suggested that age can play a role in the contagion of violence. Dr. Dubow cited that the youngest children within his studies have been the most impressionable in terms of the exposure to violence. Additionally, evidence shows that exposure to ethnopolitical violence adversely affects a child's emotional security toward his or her community, which in turn leads to more externalizing behaviors such as aggression and attention disorders (Cummings et al., 2010, 2011). Dr. Gould noted that suicide clusters occur primarily among teenagers and young adults in the United States. She commented that one of the hypotheses for the youth factor is that neurocognitive functioning in adolescence is not fully developed. Youth decision making and impulsivity might be one reason why young people may be more susceptible to transmissions through media reporting and other peer and social networks.

Socioeconomic Factors

Dr. Rosenberg noted that one of the increasing interests in global health and disease prevention is social and economic determinants, possibly even more so than physiological determinants of health. He suggested this is an area that holds great potential for contributing to the contagion of violence model. Dr. Slutkin commented that violence itself is a social and economic determinant of the other health issues and, arguably, could be the dominant social and economic determinant of health outcomes. Dr. Fagan added that the socioeconomic determinants that often are risk factors of violence are also risk factors for other adverse health outcomes.

IMPLICATIONS FOR INTERVENTION

The evidence supporting the contagion of violence within and across types of violence has implications for designing interventions to interrupt the contagion. Many speakers commented that, like other infectious diseases, a reduction in the spread of violence requires interventions that reduce susceptibility and devise new norms. Several speakers also noted that interventions designed to prevent the spread of one type of violence often have either positive or negative effects on the spread of other types of violence.

Interventions can be multidirectional. Dr. Watts cited an example of an intervention in Côte d'Ivoire that was focused on preventing intimate partner violence by working with men to redefine constructs of masculinity. In follow-up surveys, the data collected suggested that some men involved in the intervention program chose not to become involved in current ethnopolitical violence because of the experience they had during the intervention program. However, some multidirectional consequences can be negative. Dr. Fagan told an anecdote of a policing program in New York that involves stopping individuals to search for illegal guns, increasing the number of young women carrying guns because they are not stopped and searched as often as men.

Some speakers suggested that interventions should focus on changing social norms. Dr. Watts suggested that changing social norms around the construct of masculinity has been shown to prevent the contagion of family violence. She also noted that intervention programs often focus on the woman who had been a victim of intimate partner violence, but do not address the children within the household. She suggested that interventions targeted for the entire household are key to interrupting the contagion of violence. Dr. Fagan suggested that retooling the relationship between the police and gun offenders could help interrupt community-level violence. Unregulated punishment can exacerbate susceptibility to violence and increase the network density of people who share police victimization experiences. Dr. Gould commented that, to interrupt suicide contagion, social norms regarding talking openly about suicide risks need to change. There is a myth that because suicide is contagious, you cannot ask about suicide. However, you can assess for suicidal ideation without making a person think that he or she should commit suicide.

Dr. Dubow commented on the importance of interventions focused on protective factors. Most interventions to prevent ethnopolitical violence are trauma-focused. However, the evidence is showing the importance of protective factors and such interventions can be implemented in school and community settings. He also noted the importance of enhancing the protective factor of the family (specifically, the family is protective against exposure to violence on children), by bolstering the family itself. This could be through providing mental health services to families during times of ethnopolitical conflict, or in the case of reintegration post-conflict (such in the case of child soldiers), by providing extra-familial activities such as work that reduce stress on the family structure itself.

Speaker Carl Bell of the Community Mental Health Council commented that one of the challenges with public health interventions to interrupt epidemics is that the epidemics often are cyclical. He gave the example of a syphilis epidemic in gay men in Chicago: "We put signs on the buses. The epidemic went away. The signs came down. The epidemic came back." He suggested that three things are needed to stop an epidemic: an evidence base, an implementation system, and political will.

Key Messages Raised by Individual Speakers

- Violence is contagious both within and across types of violence (Dubow, Fagan, Gould, Huesmann, Slutkin, Watts).
- Social norms contribute to the contagion of violence and norms change has the potential to interrupt it (Fagan, Gould, Slutkin, Watts).
- Media can both facilitate and prevent the contagion of violence; however, the role of the Internet in the contagion process is not well understood (Fagan, Gould, Huesmann, Watts).
- Dose-response effect applies across types of violence (Dubow, Gould, Watts).
- Understanding the contagion process can inform the development of violence prevention interventions as well as illuminate potential unintended consequences that affect other types of violence (Bell, Fagan, Gould, Watts).

REFERENCES

Abramsky, T., C. Watts, C. Garcia-Moreno, K. Devries, L. Kiss, M. Ellsberg, H. Jansen, and L. Heise 2011. What factors are associated with recent intimate partner violence? Findings from the WHO multi-country study on women's health and domestic violence. *BMC Public Health* 11:109.

Crooks, C. V. 2011. The science of interrupting/preventing the cycle of violence. Presented at IOM Workshop on Preventing Violence Against Women and Children, Washington, DC, January 27.

Cummings, E. M., E. Cairns, M. C. Goeke-Morey, C. E. Merrilees, A. C. Schermerhorn, and P. Shirlow. 2010. Political violence and child adjustment in Northern Ireland: Testing pathways in a social-ecological model including single- and two-parent families. *Developmental Psychology* 46:827-841.

Cummings, E. M., E. Cairns, M. C. Goecke-Morey, C. E. Merrilees, A. C. Schermerhorn, and P. Shirlow. 2011. Longitudinal pathways between political violence and child adjustment: The role of emotional security about the community in Northern Ireland. *Journal of Abnormal Child Psychology* 39:213-224.

Devries, K., C. Watts, M. Yoshihama, L. Kiss, L. B. Schraiber, N. Deyessa, L. Heise, J. Durand, J. Mbwambo, H. Jansen, Y. Berhane, M. Ellsberg, C. Garcia-Moreno. 2011. Violence against women is strongly associated with suicide attempts: Evidence from the WHO multi-country study on women's health and domestic violence against women. *Social Science Medicine* 73(1):79-86.

Dubow, E. F., L. R. Boxer, J. Ginges, S. Gvirsman, L. R. Huesmann, S. Landau, and K. Shikaki. 2010. Exposure to conflict and violence across contexts: Relations to adjustment among Palestinian children. *Journal of Clinical Child and Adolescent Psychology* 39:103-116.

Gould, M. S. 1990. Suicide clusters and media exposure. In *Suicide over the life cycle: Risk factors, assessment, and treatment of suicidal patients*, edited by S. Blumenthal and D. Kupfer. Washington, DC: American Psychiatric Association. Pp. 517-532.

Hagihara, A., T. Abe, and K. Tarumi. 2007. Media suicide-reports: Internet use and the occurrence of suicides between 1987 and 2005 in Japan. *BMC Public Health* 11(7):321.

Kelly, S. 2010. Exposure to gang violence in the community: An integrated review of the literature. *Journal of Child and Adolescent Psychiatric Nursing* 23:61-73.

Motto, J. A. 1970. Newspaper influence on suicide. *Archives of General Psychiatry* 23:143-148.

Mullins, C. W., B. A. Jacobs, and R. Wright. 2004. Gender, streetlife and criminal retaliation. *Criminology* 42:911-940.

3

Processes and Mechanisms of the Contagion of Violence

In the previous chapter, the spread and transmission of violence was documented across individuals, groups, and generations, as well as through different ecological levels. This chapter will explore the questions of how such violence spreads and what the processes and mechanisms are of the transmission of violence.

A well-known paradigm in public health called the Haddon Matrix (see Figure 3-1), which is a model used to conceptualize injuries and injury prevention, was described by speaker Jeffrey Victoroff of the University of Southern California Keck School of Medicine. The Haddon Matrix has two axes: (1) the vertical axis is temporal, divided in pre-, peri-, and post-event; and (2) the horizontal axis is ecological, divided into personal, agent or vector, physical environment, and social environment. At the intersection of each row and column, one asks what the relevant factors are. For example, what personal factors contributed to the injury before the event? What social factors need to be considered following the event (e.g., to mitigate the effects of the injury or to prevent the injury from occurring again)? The

	Individual	Agent/Vector	Physical Environment	Social Environment
Pre-event				
Event				
Post-event				

FIGURE 3-1 Haddon Matrix.

Haddon Matrix is also a useful model to consider how different elements interact with each other, from micro to macro, and from before the event to after the event (Haddon, 1968).

Speakers on the panel on theories, processes, and mechanisms explored the contagion of violence at the macro level, including social influences and group dynamics, and at the micro level, including social-cognitive learning and neurological mechanisms. While at each level there are risk and protective factors for violence occurring and being transmitted, there are also factors that result in violence moving from one level to another. For example, several speakers noted that types of violence rarely occur alone—family violence is more prevalent in the context of community violence, and community violence can have destabilizing effects at state or national levels. The panel also explored the potential application of this discussion to possible interventions, using the knowledge presented. In explaining the importance of this, moderator Robert Ursano of the Center for the Study of Traumatic Stress of the Uniformed Services University of the Health Sciences noted several examples in which understanding the mechanism clearly maximized the impact of the most effective intervention, including child neglect in military families and reducing suicide by addressing anxiety versus depression.

Forum member and planning committee chair Rowell Huesmann of the University of Michigan noted that infectivity of violence is not limited to victimization or perpetration, but also observation of violence (including via media). This implication of a wider susceptible population means that, unlike biological contagion, the contagion of violence does not require direct contact with an agent of infection. In addition, Dr. Huesmann suggested that, because observation also increases risk, the processes resulting in violence are related to that observation. Even in being directly involved in a violent act (as a victim or a perpetrator), a person is also observing that act (Huesmann and Kirwil, 2007).

SHORT-TERM PROCESSES

In the short term, Dr. Huesmann posited, exposure to violence leads to increased risk of behaving aggressively, which is a risk factor for violence. However, as Dr. Huesmann pointed out, this is a predisposing factor to violence that would require other elements to definitively result in an act of violence. Speaker Deanna Wilkinson of The Ohio State University also addressed this point, noting that perpetrators are not violent all the time, but that they are moving through their social milieu responding to social cues; some lead to violence and some do not. She noted that determining why violence happens sometimes and not other times despite similar neurological processes occurring requires examining the external context as well.

The short-term mechanisms that Dr. Huesmann referenced include priming, mimicry, and excitation transfer (Huesmann, 1988). In priming, stimulating one part of the brain results in activation of related parts, and lowers the threshold for such activation to occur again when faced with the same or similar stimuli. Thus, being exposed to violence or an associated element causes a cascade of reactions in the brain, which is poised to process more quickly the next time it is exposed. If such a cascade results in a violent response, this same response might occur more readily in the future. Excitation transfer, Dr. Huesmann noted, is more subtle. Observation of violence increases emotional arousal, but how that is experienced depends on individual and contextual factors. However, Dr. Huesmann also noted that if such excitation is accompanied by provocation or other situation likely to result in anger, then the arousal experienced by observing violence is likely to include anger, thus heightening the excitatory response.

Mimicry and Imitation

Mimicry involves copying behavior of someone with whom one identifies. Children can learn from mimicry, so observing violence would provide examples for how others respond to specific events. Speaker Marco Iacoboni from the University of California, Los Angeles, further explored the process of mimicry. He described cells within the brain called mirror neurons, which fire both when performing certain actions and when observing others perform those same actions. In firing during observation, the brain is simulating the action as a learning mechanism. Dr. Iacoboni described such neurons in particular regions of the brain, most notably those related to motor functioning and vision and memory, as explored through emerging research. Thus, Dr. Iacoboni notes, mirror neurons fire when performing certain motor activities such as grasping a door knob, when watching another person grasp a doorknob so as to learn the action, and when recording the memory of the action. Such a process is useful in learning behavior and also in recognizing behavior immediately, without taxing the brain with complex neural processing. Dr. Iacoboni also noted that the ability of mirror neurons to mimic others' behaviors is an important element in social bonding and empathy, as well as the flip side of socially detrimental behavior of aggression and violence. For further information on the research involving imitation and mirror neurons, see Part II.

LONG-TERM PROCESSES

In the long run, Dr. Huesmann noted, violence is transmitted because observation results in changes in the cognitive functioning of the brain relevant to cues in the social environment. Specifically, the brain responds to stimuli by creating scripts, schemas, and attributions about the external environment and the individual's role within it. These processes allow the brain to develop consistent responses to repeated stimuli. If the stimuli cause intense emotional arousal, the brain's response is to become desensitized. Dr. Huesmann suggested that such an adaptation was evolutionarily advantageous so as to prevent incapacitation caused by a strong stress response.

Such schemas and scripts are created through the shorter term processes described previously, and establish consistent "shortcuts" of behavior. Those who have observed violence repeatedly, particularly violence as a response to stressful, provocative, or other emotionally charged situations, create schemas of the world in which more hostility is assumed than might truly exist. They also create scripts, like "programs" of behavior, which provide instruction on how to react to certain stimuli, primed by previous exposure, observation, and response. In situations in which hostility is attributed to the other party (whether or not the hostility exists, known as hostile attribution bias), the brain immediately processes this shortcut and retrieves the appropriate script in response.

Dr. Huesmann referred to this observational learning as a complex process potentially specific to the higher intellectual functioning of intelligent mammals, because it is not simply a biological response, but also an emotional and cognitive one. In addition, observational learning requires interpretation of others' actions as well as inferences into the meaning of others' words, actions, and thoughts.

AGGRESSION

Dr. Huesmann noted that experiencing violence increases aggression and the risk of retaliatory violence. However, he also noted that aggression itself does not always result in violence, but instead requires other precipitating factors for further violence to occur. He also noted that the attribution of aggression in others is one social cognition that plays a role in the contagion of violence.

Dr. Victoroff elaborated further on individual and collective aggression, noting that aggression is not necessarily antisocial. Dr. Victoroff noted that from an evolutionary perspective, aggression can often have an advantage, such as in cooperative hunting. Such "prosocial" aggression occurs via the same brain and social mechanisms as antisocial aggression, but has beneficial results. Aggression is also correlated with age: peaking early and then declining through life.

Dr. Victoroff also noted that collective aggression resulted in conditions favorable to the genetic success of altruism. This point was echoed later in the discussion of the hormone oxytocin and social bonding, as a result of an audience question. Though it is normally thought of as a hormone that encourages human bonding and altruism, several speakers also noted that oxytocin most likely operates by making social information more salient. So, rather than always encouraging prosocial behavior, it actually heightens existing tendencies. Speaker Jamil Zaki of Stanford University highlighted an example of someone with borderline personality disorder being less trusting under the influence of oxytocin. He also noted that oxytocin will encourage parochialism toward the members of the in-group, and potentially hostility toward the out-group. Dr. Victoroff agreed, also noting that some research shows that oxytocin increases prejudice to out-groups and nationalistic feelings for in-groups. Dr. Victoroff also indicated that such a mechanism is important in considering altruism as a potential antidote to violence because, barring grave physical threat, it is difficult to select for those individuals with a heightened tendency toward altruism.

In further exploring the notion of contagion and aggression, Dr. Victoroff posited that for such behaviors to be transmitted intergenerationally, brain structures would have to adapt and evolve, and systems would have to develop to support the various mechanisms being described. Not everyone participates in and imitates aggression, and some choose prosocial versus antisocial violence. Individuals vary as to their susceptibility to these mechanisms, and various exogenous factors influence this susceptibility. Dr. Victoroff noted that biological mechanisms might also play a role, specifically noting two brain structures involved: the ventral tegmental area and the nucleus accumbens, the latter being involved in subjective reward. He referenced studies that show differences in these brain structures in psychopaths and non-psychopaths. He also noted research showing higher basal testosterone levels in youth who were more sympathetic to terrorism than those who were not. Dr. Victoroff speculated that these exogenous and endogenous factors interacted in ways that resulted in tendency to aggression or not, and that the context in which aggression occurs plays a major role in whether such aggression leads to favorable or unfavorable outcomes. For further information on aggression and reciprocal altruism, please see Part II.

SOCIAL INTEGRATION AND REINFORCEMENT LEARNING

Dr. Zaki further examined the neurobiological processes of contagion through his discussion of social integration and the structures of the brain associated with rewards. Dr. Zaki noted that rewards are an important motivator for human behavior, both in that they are indicators of positive outcomes and that people actively seek out rewards. Rewards are essential in reinforcement learning to strengthen a desired behavior. He pointed out that not all rewards are material, and that social scientists have long regarded social integration as a type of reward (Baumeister and Leary, 1995).

Dr. Zaki noted that reinforcement learning has two essential elements: (1) prediction of reward, and (2) adaptation. While the brain responds to rewards, it eventually learns to predict when such rewards occur by identifying social and other temporal cues preceding the presentation of a reward (O'Doherty et al., 2003). A well-known example of this is Pavlov's experiments in which dogs identified the ringing of a bell with a reward of a treat. What is noteworthy in this, Dr. Zaki points out, is that the brain eventually stops responding to the reward itself and instead responds to the predictor of the reward. This response occurs in the nucleus accumbens. In addition to predicting rewards, people adapt behavior in order to actively gain rewards. Often this adaptation occurs in ways in which people do not necessarily understand.

Given this, Dr. Zaki posited that one predictor of the reward of social integration is consensus with other people. This indicates that an individual will not only respond to agreement with other people, but will also actively seek such conformity, even to the point of changing their own behavior. Dr. Zaki demonstrated through research that this seems to be the case, both psychologically and neurologically. In one such study, participants were asked to rate attractiveness of various faces. They were then told the ratings their peers gave. Upon being asked to rate the faces again, the responses of the participants changed, at a statistically significant level, so as to conform to the opinions of their peers. He also noted that this change occurred not just at a superficial level, but also at a deeper level in which participants truly believed in their new opinions, as observed by viewing whether the structures of the brain responding to facial attractiveness were activated (Zaki et al., 2011). Dr. Zaki speculated that, given the power of this mechanism, reinforcement learning could indicate that those in situations of high violence might be internalizing their attempts at conformity. Over time, this may lead to intractability. He also noted, however, that research indicates this mechanism is very generalizable, and it would be useful to consider how it could be used to promote the spread of prosocial behavior.

GROUP DYNAMICS

Psychological and physiological processes within individuals have the potential to shed light on the mechanism of the contagion of violence. Speakers also noted the importance of such processes interacting with the context or environment in which stimuli, observation, and conformity occur. Other speakers considered the importance of that context or environment itself, as well as the interplay of multiple factors. In particular, the role of group dynamics, alluded to previously in terms of collective aggression, altruism, and conformity, has a synergistic effect with the role of neurobiology in influencing decision making.

Dr. Wilkinson explored the mechanism of group dynamics and its role in the contagion of violence. She echoed the comments of several speakers in noting the importance of schemas, scripts, attribution, collective responsibility, conformity, and imitation, and explored these within the context of group violence. In particular, she noted the strong influence of peers and an individual's reputation.

Group affiliation, such as in gangs, is correlated with increased risk of violence, as victim, perpetrator, or witness. Often, these groups exist within a social ecology in which allegiance is seen as protective against outside danger (Wilkinson and Carr, 2008). As previously noted, youth create their identities through observational learning and socialization, and much of the violence that occurs within groups is public. Dr. Wilkinson especially noted that expectations of behavior are created collectively, versus individually. This is more than peer pressure, she argues, but also a diffusion of responsibility throughout the group. Thus, social integration brings with it the scripts and schemas that underlie behavior.

In unpacking the violent event, Dr. Wilkinson noted that in her research she was very interested in knowing what was occurring in the participants' minds, and also in the co-occurrences of the event. In one study of hers, she noted two major additional factors: (1) the presence of a third party, and (2) the gossip that occurs before and after the event. Both speak to peers and reputation, and the status of the antagonists and protagonists within the group. She also pointed out the implication of retaliation, which she noted occurred about one third of the time. From this research, she posits five types of peer group influence related to violence, with implications for why violence spreads:

1. Planning involvement in advance
2. Coming to the aid of an associate who is losing
3. Being an observer who is threatened during the interaction
4. Seeking justice or righting a perceived wrong
5. Addressing gossip to protect reputation

Social Influence and Intersectionality

At the macro level, factors within society influence not only how and when violence occurs, but also how it might be transmitted. Speaker Anita Raj of the University of California, San Diego, discussed the interaction of multiple social factors in the context of intimate partner violence. She noted that her original research in HIV prevention indicated that expectations of behavior based solely on social-cognitive models would not always

accurately predict outcome because of the influence of other intersection-
alities, both within a community and a larger, national, or global scale. In
particular, one major impact on the risk of intimate partner violence is the
role of gender inequality and race. But, despite interventions that might
seek to empower women, violence might not necessarily be reduced because of the other contextual factors involving perpetrators, norms around
behavior, other inequities such as lack of education or increased substance
abuse, and other structural issues. Dr. Raj also the noted the importance
of moving upstream and thinking about interventions that address larger
social issues such as incarceration and homelessness.

In thinking about an ecological framework within which to explore
intimate partner violence, Dr. Raj also noted the importance of addressing
"biology, behavior, state." The first is the physiological or neurological
processes that might be occurring at the individual level, as noted by other
speakers. The second might include comorbidities such as substance abuse
or risk-taking behavior. The third might include mental health. Also at the
individual level, she highlighted the importance of gender equality in the
context of the relationship (versus as a social norm) as a possible point of
interruption. She also highlighted the importance of family norms, particularly in the context of reinforcement learning, noting how certain violent
behaviors might lead to a favorable outcome and no repercussions; and in
observational learning, children modeling parents' behavior as socialization. She closed on the importance of understanding that the acceptability
of violence is also transmitted through generations and across communities.

INTERRUPTING THE TRANSMISSION OF VIOLENCE

In thinking about how violence is transmitted across the ecological dimensions, through generations, and from individual to individual, speakers
also examined the possibility for interruption. Dr. Ursano stated that not
all interventions present themselves so readily:

> But we must keep in mind that strep throat is not a penicillin deficiency
> and yet penicillin is a marvelous intervention for the infection of strep.
> Similarly perhaps the most important psychological intervention ever in-
> vented is in fact the seatbelt because the seatbelt prevents a psychiatric
> illness. It prevents posttraumatic stress disorder (PTSD) because people
> who are injured are at four times greater risk of developing PTSD. As we
> begin to think from mechanisms to interventions, we are going to have to
> take on several different lenses to be able to accomplish that.

Dr. Raj noted several interventions in her presentation designed to
prevent violence specifically, but with applicability for interruption as well,
as they focus on the transmission of social norms. She also noted some

interventions that focused on mitigating factors, such as unemployment or reproductive coercion, which could have an impact on vulnerability. She mentioned the importance of looking at interventions which, while intending to address one type of violence, might have the benefit of addressing other types of violence as well, further highlighting the interaction of multiple forms of violence.

Speakers also hypothesized, based on the information presented, possible types of interventions that might be successful. Dr. Huesmann speculated that inoculating children against developing negative schemas and scripts and instead teaching prosocial and compassionate scripts would result in decreased uptake of observed violence. However, he noted the issue of not preventing emotional dysregulation that would still naturally occur because of the exposure to violence. Dr. Wilkinson suggested that programs that intervene in social situations in which isolation and lack of opportunity occur have proven to be very successful; she cited Cure Violence (formerly known as CeaseFire) as an example. Dr. Raj noted that, given the role of modeling and mirror neurons described by Dr. Iacoboni, being able to provide positive role models to emulate would be essential. She advocated for putting further effort into identifying such positive role models, as well as confronting the structural issues that lead to the removal of such models from communities. Dr. Victoroff found that giving men the opportunity to be a provider and get married would reduce their likelihood of joining terrorist cells, and he speculated this could apply to other group affiliations. Several others cautioned that marriage, while being beneficial for men, is not always beneficial for women, so it would be important not to unintentionally increase risk of other types of violence. Dr. Zaki reiterated the potentially powerful use of social conformity, and indicated that one possible approach would be—through social network analysis—to identify the most influential individual in a group or community and change his or her behavior or norms, with the expectation of uptake of that change throughout the group. Dr. Iacoboni noted that even though mirror neurons might fire, people do not constantly mimic each other, so some measure of self-control is being exerted. He suggested exploring the idea of an intervention that could augment self-control.

Participants also explored further application of their ideas in discussing interventions that might reduce social isolation or might increase integration among groups. Dr. Zaki speculated that breaking down barriers between groups could increase prosocial behavior toward those not part of the in-group. He also noted that identities are generally flexible. It is possible to consider oneself part of a very narrow group and also as part of a larger group at any given time. He cited a study in which fans of two soccer teams expressed hostility toward each other when discussing their own teams, but when discussing soccer in general were complimentary toward each other and somewhat hostile toward non-soccer fans. He noted that one thing that creates an in-group is having an out-group as a counterpoint, and wondered if it would be possible to create a large enough group identity to include everyone. Dr. Huesmann noted that one way to reduce barriers between groups is to have them believe they are more alike than unalike.

Speakers and audience members also challenged assumptions about violence and its contagion. In response to an audience member's question about why violence is not always contagious, Dr. Raj brought up the notion of positive deviance. Dr. Wilkinson noted that people are not divided into "violent" and "nonviolent," but that violence is emergent from situations. She also emphasized that violence is functional, and is not always the response that will garner the most advantageous outcome. She urged additional research into why siblings exposed to similar factors will not all end up committing or being a victim of violence. Dr. Ursano summarized these thoughts with proposing the idea of thinking about "absence of violence as deviance." Speaker and planning committee member Gary Slutkin of the University of Illinois at Chicago closed the discussion by commenting on the possibility that infection still occurs at high rates, but few actually develop the syndrome.

Key Messages as Noted by Individual Speakers

- It is important to take into account complex interaction of social and biological factors (Raj, Ursano, Wilkinson, Zaki).
- It would be illuminating to further explore how violence is not contagious (Iacoboni, Raj, Ursano, Wilkinson) and how non-violence can be contagious (Victoroff, Zaki).
- Multiple processes within the brain could explain physiological changes resulting in increased risk of violence (Huesmann, Iacoboni, Victoroff, Zaki).
- Important social processes and group dynamics could explain increase risk of violence (Huesmann, Raj, Wilkinson, Zaki).
- The interruption of violence could be explored not only from the perspective of proximal causes and effects, but also thinking about upstream or more distal factors (Iacoboni, Raj, Ursano).

REFERENCES

Baumeister, R. F., and M. R. Leary. 1995. The need to belong: Desire for interpersonal attachments as a fundamental human-motivation. *Psychological Bulletin* 117(3):497-529.
Haddon, W., Jr. 1968. The changing approach to the epidemiology, prevention, and amelioration of trauma: The transition to approaches etiologically rather than descriptively based. *American Journal of Public Health and the Nation's Health* 58(8):1431-1438.

Huesmann, L. R. 1988. An information-processing model for the development of aggression. *Aggressive Behavior* 14(1):13-24.

Huesmann, L. R., and L. Kirwil. 2007. Why observing violence increases the risk of violent behavior in the observer. In *The Cambridge handbook of violent behavior and aggression*, edited by D. Flannery. Cambridge, UK: Cambridge University Press.

O'Doherty, J. P., P. Dayan, K. Friston, H. Critchley, and R. J. Dolan. 2003. Temporal difference models and reward-related learning in the human brain. *Neuron* 38(2):329-337.

Wilkinson, D. L., and P. J. Carr. 2008. Violent youths' responses to high levels of exposure to community violence: What violent events reveal about youth violence. *Journal of Community Psychology* 36(8):1026-1051.

Zaki, J., J. Schirmer, and J. P. Mitchell. 2011. Social influence modulates the neural computation of value. *Psychological Science* 22(7):894-900.

4

The Role of Contextual Factors in the Contagion of Violence

INTRODUCTION

For violence to infect, certain individual, social, and environmental factors must be present. The previous chapter explored some of the individual and social mechanisms that might explain the contagion of violence. This chapter explores some of the contextual factors that might moderate the contagion. The individual and group mechanisms that provide the pathway from observation to perpetration of violence can be mediated by a number of additional elements; such a constellation of factors and circumstances vary from individual to individual and from population to population, and vary across types and modes of violence.

In the fourth session of the workshop, mediators and cofactors that affect risk of and resilience to the spread of violence were discussed. Speakers in this session highlighted some factors that create the synergistic formula that enables the infectivity of violence across cultures, groups, and types of violence. To be susceptible or immune to violence, the "right" constellation of factors need to be present or absent. This chapter focuses on such factors with respect to systems and practices that contribute to the exacerbation, reduction, or prevention of violence, leveraging the classic epidemiologic model of infectious disease: spread, susceptibility, and immunity.

FACTORS THAT PROMOTE OR HINDER SUSCEPTIBILITY

Most relevant to this concept of the contagious nature of violence is the vulnerability or susceptibility of individuals and communities to violence and to the transmission of violence. There are important contextual factors within communities, such as who are marginalized or culturally isolated and who have normalized violence, and certain risk factors that accompany violence, such as alcohol and drugs. The speakers used contextual factors to frame the discussion of violence within the contagion framework.

Place

Many speakers noted that place can have adverse impacts on health. The context in which violence occurs determines proximity to exposure, and how often a person is exposed (similar to dose). The place in which violence occurs also influences whether an individual sees violence as a "normal" response, whether they have resources that could counter violence, and whether they have opportunities to respond without violence.

Speaker Barry Krisberg of the University of California, Berkeley, School of Law spoke about place in terms of the experience of prison that "produces a whole series of dysfunctional, psychological developments." He showed two photographs of a California treatment facility, stating, "The youth who stays in this facility has committed a violent crime, and he spends 21 hours a day in this room, getting all kinds of cognitive behavioral therapy, but this is his life. When he is fortunate enough to get out, for an hour or so, he gets to exercise in this, which is described euphemistically as his program area. . . . This is fairly typical. In fact, unless you live in the state of Missouri, your facilities look pretty much this way."

Dr. Krisberg noted that many believe that if we make prison so horrible, people will avoid committing violence to stay out of these places. In addition, taking offenders "out of circulation," or incapacitation, means that they are not "on the street" committing crime. On the contrary, Dr. Krisberg stated, prisons and juvenile facilities exacerbate and spread violence. They are much more violent than the general community, and the perpetrators of violence in prison are both staff and inmates. Much of the violence in prison is related to gangs, and the experience of being a victim increases the risk of joining a gang, which further cements these gang structures (Wolff and Shi, 2009). Dr. Krisberg went on to comment that who actually commits violence in prison is not clear. It is not necessarily true that those who commit violence outside prison are those who are most violent in prison. However, those with histories of assault and robbery (though not homicide) are at increased risk of perpetration of violence while incarcerated.

In terms of the psychological effects of incarceration, Dr. Krisberg brought up the previously hypothesized idea of "prisonization" or institutionalization, in which one adapts or develops an inmate culture or ideal. This has changed slightly, Dr. Krisberg stated, but in general, "prisons promulgate a view of the world, and inmates are expected to adopt that view of the world. It is not a view of the world that is particularly helpful if you are trying to live a successful, peaceful life."

Another important element of place is transition across places—such as community to prison and then back to the community. Dr. Krisberg noted that 700,000 people exit American prisons every year. Of those, 93 percent return home, most of them within 3 years (West, 2008). Within 3 years, 67 percent of returning prisoners were rearrested for serious offenses, and 52 percent were returned to prison for new criminal offenses (Langan and Levin, 2002), though homicide and sexual offenders had the lowest rates of recidivism. However, released prisoners in general commit a lot of crime in the community. A 1990 study by the Department of Justice shows that released prisoners have a homicide rate 53 times that of the general population. Dr. Krisberg urged that further research on the dynamics of prisons was warranted, to understand how they might exacerbate the spread of violence, versus serving as "deterrent mechanisms."

Another layer of the complexity of place as a contextual factor is the aging population of prisoners. Dr. Krisberg mentioned that a large percentage of prisoners are older adults—approximately 30 to 40 percent of prisoners are over age 55—and there is some suggestion that older inmates are victimized by younger ones. If violence and exploitation are central to the institution, vulnerable populations, such as older inmates, may suffer disproportionately, especially as their faculties deteriorate.

Dr. Krisberg also spoke of place in terms of juvenile justice facilities. There are studies focused on juvenile facilities suggesting that 45 to 72 percent of youth released from juvenile facilities are committing new crimes. He also stated that there is a strong body of research that indicates that placing low-level juvenile offenders in correctional facilities (versus leaving them in the community) increases recidivism and school failure, among other measures. Incarceration for youth traditionally is viewed as a social work intervention, especially in the context of bad living situations or neighborhood and family environments. But research in Florida and other places show that incarceration for youth increases risk of violence and other adverse outcomes, mainly due to peer influences (Baglivio, 2007).

Dr. Krisberg used an example to illustrate the role of place with respect to the contagion of violence. He commented on a study performed 40 years ago by Phillip Zombardo of Stanford University in which a group of Stanford students were randomly assigned, with some students as inmates and some as guards. A dormitory was converted into a mock prison. Within 3 days, the experiment was halted because several of the Stanford students who were assigned to be inmates were showing serious mental health symptoms, some as serious as psychosis. The Stanford students who were the guards were manifesting vicious, violent, and assaultive behavior against the so-called inmates. Dr. Krisberg stated, "Here are well-educated, upper class, primarily white students, who were put in the crudest form of role playing around prisons. Yet, it immediately [and] dramatically increased the level of violence, both [among] the students [who played the role of prisoners] and the ones who played the role of guards."

Another example of contagion is clear with the growing body of research indicating that people leave prison with potential for increased rates of partner violence and child abuse. Speaker Deborah Gorman-Smith of Chapin Hall at the University of Chicago stated that "we see the contagion passing onto the next generation. As prisoners coming out take out this anger and frustration on their family members, it creates the breeding ground for an intergenerational transfer of violence" (White et al., 2002; Oliver and Hairston, 2008). Dr. Gorman-Smith applauded the fact that there is currently one of the most dramatic decarcerations in American history, as the rate of juvenile incarceration decreases, and there is a national trend to close juvenile justice facilities.

Another important consideration of place that Speaker Fariyal Ross-Sheriff of Howard University mentioned is the role of migration and displacement. Dr. Ross-Sheriff discussed violence during preuprooting, uprooting, and transition stages, and she spoke of the stages that are considered safe and protective factors and contribute to resilience.

In terms of the stages of migration, Dr. Ross-Sheriff spoke of the most difficult time as the preuprooting stage, which is considered to be between 1 year and 6 weeks before a person or group decides to leave. She then spoke of the transition stage, such as in refugee camps and countries of first asylum. She stated that despite the effort on the part of the first country of asylum to provide support, resettlement only tends to occur in the second country of asylum. In terms of intervention opportunities, Dr. Ross-Sheriff stated that "resettlement and adaptation in host societies are the times when we can provide services, when we can make differences."

But, violence is often committed by many groups who are charged with protecting refugees, including soldiers, police, and others, such as administrators, camp staff, and other refugees. "Violence occurs for many, many women who are trying to deal with their day-to-day survival and livelihood, just for getting food, for trying to bring water, to get fuel." Violence can also occur within the home, "if the spouse or the family finds out that the woman has been raped, then she is used property. She goes through now more problems at home."

Poverty

Another important contextual factor is poverty, especially with respect to marginalized and impoverished communities. Poverty, as a conduit of such things as hopelessness, economic repression, fear, lack of resources, and isolation, create an ideal breeding ground for the promulgation of violence. For example, Dr. Iris PrettyPaint of Native Aspirations commented that Native Americans do not understand what is meant by "recession" because, for them, it is the norm, sometimes experiencing well over 40 percent unemployment. She also commented that Native Americans are wards of the government, which creates economic dependency. She stated that needing to depend on someone else can be devastating to people.

Culture and Cultural Context

Dr. PrettyPaint summarized the importance of embracing culture in this work, saying "When the cultural context comes into your work . . . it is going to be very natural for you to create things that are beneficial to any culture of people. But you leave out one of them, and you run the risk of people being confused." Dr. PrettyPaint emphasized that culture confers certain worldviews and norms that need to be heeded.

For example, Native people, especially the elders, view violence as rooted in their own cultural constructs and language of what violence means and represents, and how it impacts their communities. Dr. PrettyPaint stated that when asking Native elders to reflect on violence as contagious they stated that violence was "dangerous . . . we need to find the medicine to heal someone from this [contagion of violence] or protect them from it." She further noted, "if you communicate that [violence] is incurable, that is not something that I think is in their worldview. [Native elders] don't believe that; they think there is something somewhere that they can find [to heal it]."

When cultural practices and traditions are removed from the environment of communities and individuals, then violence has a greater chance of causing infection. With respect to Native children, Dr. PrettyPaint emphasized that a journey of forced assimilation creates an environment that helps nurture violence in them. She stated, "these children have lost their ability to know who they are, and they have multiple identities." When children are removed from their culture, they lose their place or context. Dr. PrettyPaint emphasized the importance of examining the integrity of cultural practices for violence prevention. "Today, we have young people that are relearning how to speak their language. We have tribes that are rewriting their constitutions to open up an enrollment process so that all children living in their community can be enrolled and eligible for health care [and] education." Thus, this connection to culture and cultural practices helps create a place or meaningful connection of an individual to a greater whole. Such connection creates an environment in which there can be reduced transmission of violence.

Historical Oppression and Trauma

Dr. PrettyPaint further spoke about historical trauma in the context of the contagion of violence, noting that historical trauma creates a cumulative emotional, psychological, and physical insult on individuals and communities and increases one's vulnerability to violence. The perspective of historical trauma is critical to understanding the ability of violence to infect susceptible individuals who have experienced such trauma. She stated, "I have come to recognize . . . that we have internalized the oppression and discrimination, and we have allotted lateral violence. We don't have to worry about somebody from the outside hurting us; we hurt each other."

The historical oppression of Native American people, which has been well documented, has created an environment that decreases freedoms and increases confinement, which increases the infectivity or propensity for violence. For example, Dr. PrettyPaint spoke about the lack of sovereignty:

> colonization is real, it is still alive today, and it is something that, if you haven't experienced, then it is very hard to feel it. . . . And when you don't think someone is human, then it is easy to dehumanize people. And when you do that, what you do is a form of violence, because you take away the ability for someone to speak. We know that in our way of life, the language is the key that unlocks the foundation to our worldview. Without language, you will be challenged to find meaning. You will be challenged to understand what it feels like.

Race and Racism

Dr. Ross-Sheriff mentioned the importance of intersectionality and related theories as being important to achieve a more comprehensive and balanced understanding of susceptibility to violence. "It is the intersectionality of race, gender, nationality, religion, poverty, and status of marginalization that make a difference . . . and I don't mean to say racism from the whites. Racism in Kenya can come from blacks against blacks; [e.g.,] in South Africa, the whole issue of South Africans perpetrating violence against African refugees from other places."

Racism as an act of oppression can deter resilience and immunity. There are crosscutting areas of oppression that are integral to understanding the contagion of violence. Speaker Carl Bell of Community Mental Health Council in Chicago discussed how marginalization of African American males by the U.S. criminal justice system (which reduces their ability to become resilient to or immune to violence) exacerbates their susceptibility to violence.

Gender

Dr. Gorman-Smith commented on gender and its relation to family and disruption, noting that 92 percent of incarcerated parents are men, and the number is growing. She stated that there is a lot of attention to reentry programs, but that most of those programs are focused on work and education. Dr. Gorman-Smith also noted that there are almost no programs and no single evidence-based intervention focused on helping men reenter their families as they come back from prison. Some data show that assuming an active fathering role relates to more successful reentry given that active fathering reduces depression, increases employment stability, and relates to decreased recidivism.

Dr. Ross-Sheriff spoke of resilience among migrant women who are highly impacted by violence, and out of the approximate 15-20 million global refugees (not including internally displaced people) per year, 80 percent of the refugees in refugee camps are women and children. Dr. Ross-Sheriff stated that these women and children experience physical, sexual, and emotional violence in camps, in outside spaces, and within their homes.

Mental Illness and Disabilities

Dr. Krisberg commented on the presence of mental illness and disabilities with respect to increasing an individual's susceptibility to violence. He stated that victims of violence in prisons are highly likely to be mentally ill or have cognitive or physical disabilities. Such disabilities can add increased stress and trauma in an already violent environment.

Family

Dr. Gorman-Smith spoke about social and structural moderators with respect to the role of family and positive parenting. She stated that families are central to understanding violence and the contagion. Dr. Gorman-Smith listed important aspects of parenting and family functioning that can increase susceptibility to violence, aggression in youth, family and intimate partner violence, and child abuse and neglect. These include various aspects of parenting practices such as harsh or coercive discipline over the course of the child's life, hostility within the family, conflict, absence of warmth or connection among family members, disruptions, family instability, having multiple partners, chaos, and multiple moves.

Dr. PrettyPaint commented on the ecological levels of family and the community as being interconnected, and thus each level influences the other. It is important, she noted, that in thinking about family, one is also thinking about community. Dr. Gorman-Smith concurred and spoke about the varying developmental spectrum of influence of families on child development, which impacts what course of action families need to take in relation to important contextual changes. She noted that it is not the case that all dysfunctional families are in violent neighborhoods, and all functional families are in safe neighborhoods, but instead types of families are more or less evenly spread across types of communities. While context plays an important role, optimally, she stated that there is a combination of parenting practices and family relationship characteristics that include emotional warmth and connection, good organizational structure, strong support belief for the families, good discipline practices, and monitoring where children are; these characteristics are important regardless of setting. But parents are also managing peers and schools, interacting with others in the neighborhood, and often dealing with issues caused by concentrated poverty and a poorly built environment. Even optimal parenting might not reduce a child's exposure to violence, so approaches to building resiliency might be required.

Forum member XinQi Dong of the Rush University Medical Center in Chicago added another dimension to the discussion of family by noting that often families, including grandparents, take on larger roles if one or more parent is missing. He questioned the impact on the grandparents: whether the stress of stepping back into the parental role might increase their own vulnerability to family violence (or suicide), and how the contagion of violence might apply to the spread of violence within the family to include elder abuse. Dr. PrettyPaint noted that in Native American communities, grandparents are often forced into the role of caring for young children, even as they age and become vulnerable themselves. Dr. Ross-Sheriff reflected that in Asian populations, elderly people experience abuse and neglect because of intergenerational conflicts, often exacerbated by the involuntary caring of grandchildren or by the inability to live independently of their own children.

IMMUNITY AND RESILIENCE

In this infectious disease framework, resilience to violence can be thought of as immunity. Within immunity and resilience, concepts of culture, place, religion, family, and the law play a role.

The Role of Culture in Building Resilience

Dr. Bell spoke about resilience with an example of South Asians in Durban, South Africa, where they are protected by their culture, which engages them in social and emotional skills and monitoring their children. He noted a similar mechanism with children of immigrants who lost the protective factors that social fabric conveys. He noted his work with the Illinois Department of Children and Family Services, which showed that when children who are victimized by violence are taught social-emotional skills and affect regulation, as well as life skills and hard work experience as positive motivation, traumatic symptoms are reduced. However, Dr. Bell also cautioned that "culture does protect, but culture also destroys," in noting how black males face disproportionately higher rates of incarceration than white males because of a propensity to closer living arrangements.

Dr. PrettyPaint spoke of "miracle survivors," noting that resilience is not necessarily taught, but can be emergent in the proper nurturing environment. The strength of Native storytelling is that it allows survivors to teach the lessons learned from violent experiences and relate them to the traditional healing practices (including song, dance, and traditional ceremonies) that exist in the culture. She described a successful Native American–focused intervention, called Native Aspirations, in Spokane, Washington. Native Aspirations empowers youth in the community with a sense of belonging and identity by providing training and technical assistance to enhance sustainable violence prevention. The program operates from the understanding that overcoming oppression is a first step toward empowerment, and imbues individuals and communities with a sense of planning and forward direction. Dr. PrettyPaint emphasized that there is not a one-size-fits-all approach and that it is possible to give data and a model to various communities, but the communities themselves need to reconstruct the program to fit the community.

Dr. Krisberg concurred that cultural context is very important when considering the contagion of violence and violence prevention programs. He emphasized the growing U.S. Latino population that is incarcerated, and noted that little research covers Latino communities and that most evidence-based programming has little understanding of cultural context.

The Role of Family in Building Resilience

Dr. Gorman-Smith highlighted family as being protective and promotive. She stated that when trying to change community-level contextual factors, it is important to also support families. Examples raised of changing context include Cure Violence (formerly known as CeaseFire) and Communities that Care, which help support the larger social environment, while working to change family functioning. Examples of impact on families include Dr. Gorman-Smith's intervention, Schools and Families Educating Children, which is an intervention delivered to all children in a neighborhood. It is delivered during first grade and uses multiple family groups, focused on issues such as discipline and monitoring, but within the context of managing the ecological niche of the neighborhoods where they live. She noted data that show an effect on the developmental trajectory through the change in parenting. She also described how the program has evidence of improved academic performance, particularly because of an emphasis of linking families and schools. The second family-level intervention she used was from the multisite study of GREAT Schools and Families. This family-focused intervention not only found effects on the aggressive kids, but also on ecological effects at the school level, with increasing divergence over time.

Forum member Clare Anderson of the Administration on Children, Youth and Families noted that a number of interventions exist for children who have experienced violence and trauma, especially to increase self-regulation, augment self-control, and create different scripts for viewing the world—and such interventions need greater uptake. The majority of these interventions include parenting elements, as well as the creation of nurturing environments.

Place/Setting as Protective

In addition to being potentially harmful, place can also be protective. Dr. Ross-Sheriff spoke of protective factors and spaces, noting that the safe spaces for refugee women are health clinics and schools, which are venues for education or training, connecting with others of shared experience, and even healing. Another protective space in terms of first countries of asylum is at houses of worship and religious community gatherings, with women who have similar experiences. After resettlement, houses of worship, social workers, and resettlement program leaders can also be helpful.

Dr. Krisberg noted changes in operations of juvenile facilities in states such as Missouri, where the intention is to create small communities where nonviolence is the norm, and life is as "normal" as possible. Some facilities are also exploring the effectiveness of having the youth create their own rules and abide by them, creating a more empowering inclusive dynamic, instead of "us versus them," and separating the youth from the violent subculture of prisons.

The Role of Law

Laws play a role in how violence is dealt with in settings such as prisons and thus create or do not create rules that protect susceptible persons. Dr. Krisberg mentioned the U.S. Prison Rape Elimination Act and the Civil Rights of Institutionalized Persons Act as examples of such laws, and also noted that the Americans with Disabilities Act is probably the single most important piece of legislation used to challenge these situations. Dr. PrettyPaint noted the complex role that jurisdiction plays in Native populations, especially because many issues of violence and crime are addressed at federal levels. She also cautioned that while laws are useful (e.g., elder justice and laws that protect elders from abuse), more work is still needed to create safe spaces for survivors to talk about the violence and trauma.

Connectedness and Community

Dr. Bell spoke of connecting youth and giving them "connectedness"; to this end, schools have a huge role as protective factors in terms of building resilience and immunity to violence. Another protective factor is the community. The importance of building and enhancing community and breaking down institutional racism within the police force and justice system are essential. He also emphasized the need to elevate the moral authority of communities, and the need to consider the negative and positive consequences on violence of the Internet and social media. While the negatives might include cyberbullying, he argued that the Internet provides opportunities to have relationships and engage in activities off the street. Dr. Ross-Sheriff agreed that technology such as mobile phones can play an important role, especially in connecting women with other female family members who might live elsewhere. Dr. Gorman-Smith noted that for children who lack warm, supportive environments at home, the collective efficacy of a stable community could promote resilience in the face of exposure to violence.

SUGGESTED RESEARCH OPPORTUNITIES

To move toward policy and practice being informed by research, the workshop speakers cited opportunities to focus future research. Forum and planning committee member Evelyn Tomaszewski of the National Association of Social Workers emphasized the importance of connecting context to the research. Dr. Krisberg stated that the variable of incarceration, including its duration and intensity, should be incorporated into longitudinal research. Dr. Gorman-Smith also emphasized examination of middle childhood in terms of optimal interventions that work to reduce risk of violence and prevention. Dr. Ross-Sheriff stated that three types of research are needed: (1) policy research in refugee camps and with refugee populations; (2) research on the second generation, specifically, those within the United States who are resettled refugees; and (3) examination of practice evidence. Dr. PrettyPaint commented that more research should incorporate evidence- and culture-based research, both qualitative and quantitative, and that indigenous researchers should be used. Dr. Ross-Sheriff concurred, and also noted it is important for future research to move from qualitative to mixed-methods research. Forum co-chair Mark Rosenberg of the Task Force for Global Health posed important questions that remain to be answered: "We talked about the notion of immunization. Are there some times when exposure to violence will protect people? When does it not protect, but when does it produce a disease, and what is the length of protection? Is there anything such as lifelong immunity? We talked about herd immunity, can it really be produced in the area of violence?"

Theresa Kilbane from the United Nations Children's Fund (UNICEF) raised the issue of experience in building the evidence base for these interventions internationally. Dr. Gorman-Smith responded that dissemination and implementation work needs to be done with current interventions and moving them to a different context. She also emphasized that there are opportunities for natural experiments with policies that are already existent in communities, and to consider different types of outcome measures.

In taking into account the public health approach using a context-informed, ecological model that leverages the framework of infectious disease to apply to the contagion of violence, a delineation of social and structural moderators and cofactors should be considered when thinking about the exacerbation, reduction, prevention, or transmission of violence. Context and the intersectionality of contexts play a strong role in this, as does culture, race, gender, politics, historical oppression, and trauma.

Key Message Raised by Individual Speakers

- Moderators of the contagion of violence have influence in multiple spheres of the ecological framework; they also can move from level to level (Gorman-Smith, PrettyPaint).
- Resilience requires attention to holistic, contextual experiences (Bell, PrettyPaint, Ross-Sheriff).
- Contextual factors have the potential for both mitigating and exacerbating the spread of violence (Bell, Gorman-Smith, Krisberg, Tomaszewski).
- Culture is a factor that can either mitigate or exacerbate the spread of violence, and influences the effectiveness of interventions (Bell, Krisberg, PrettyPaint).

REFERENCES

Baglivio, M. T., 2007. *The prediction of risk to recidivate among a juvenile offending population*, Doctoral Dissertation, University of Florida. www.djj.state.fl.us/OPA/ptassistance/documents/Dissertation.pdf (accessed August 1, 2012).

Langan, P. A., and D. J. Levin. 2002. Recidivism of prisoners released in 1994. In *Special report/Bureau of Justice Statistics*. Washington, DC: Bureau of Justice Statistics. http://purl.access.gpo.gov/GPO/LPS33477 (accessed August 1, 2012).

Oliver, W., and C. F. Hairston. 2008. Intimate partner violence during the transition from prison to the community: Perspectives of incarcerated African American men. *Journal of Aggression, Maltreatment & Trauma* 16(3):258-276.

West, H. C. 2008. *Prisoners in 2007, Bulletin/U.S. Bureau of Justice Statistics*. Washington, DC: Bureau of Justice Statistics, U.S. Department of Justice.

White, R. J., E. W. Gondolf, D. U. Robertson, B. J. Goodwin, and L. E. Caraveo. 2002. Extent and characteristics of woman batterers among federal inmates. *International Journal of Offender Therapy and Comparative Criminology* 46(4):412-426.

Wolff, N., and J. Shi. 2009. Contextualization of physical and sexual assault in male prisons: Incidents and their aftermath. *Journal of Correctional Health Care* 15(1):58-77.

5

Contagion and Interruption in Practice

The previous chapters explored the contagion of violence in the context of the pattern of spread, the possible mechanisms at both the individual and social levels, and the factors that might reduce or exacerbate exposure and transmission. Drawing from this framework, speakers also examined potential processes of interruption or mitigation. Speakers at the workshop also explored some real-life examples of this contagion at work, bringing all of these concepts together, as well as interventions currently in practice that seek to reduce it.

THE CONTAGION IN ACTION

Speakers Jason Featherstone of Surviving Our Streets and Zainab Al-Suwaij of the American-Islamic Congress both spoke of recent occurrences in which single acts of violence sparked an epidemic in very different ways.

UK Riots

On August 4, 2011, Mark Duggan was shot and killed by police in the Tottenham neighborhood of North East London, England. Two days later, friends and family marched to the police station to obtain information regarding the shooting. After several hours of silence, patience ran out, and a series of altercations led to the overturning and burning of several police cars. Captured on video, the burning cars became a symbol for those who felt frustration around relationships with law enforcement, the current

economic climate, and various political austerity measures related to education and public services. In addition, Mr. Featherstone noted, residents of
Tottenham had a preexisting ingrained mistrust of law enforcement, related
to perceived injustices and deaths in police custody over the previous decade. Mr. Featherstone also showed several video clips and commented on
the sense of relief and anticipation expressed by participants of the violent
acts that followed the initial event. Notably, many of the organizers and
participants belonged to groups with traditional rivalries, which were set
aside in these events. Following the burning of the cars, violence spread
throughout Tottenham, London, and then other parts of the United Kingdom over the next several days. Mr. Featherstone noted that rioters were
diverse and did not fit the "traditional" image.

Calls to commit violence were sent via social media to those within
close geographical proximity as well as those in other locations outside the
United Kingdom. Footage of the rioting and looting was shown constantly
on television, and made headlines in major newspapers. Violence spread
through the country for 5 days, and then subsided as police presence in the
streets ramped up significantly, and large numbers of arrests were recorded.

Through video clips and his own reflections, Mr. Featherstone painted
a complex story of not just violence throughout the country, but a sense of
resentment, frustration, and inequality that had bubbled over. Previously
that year, large antiausterity protests had been held, with little to no relief
presented. In one map he showed, there was strong geographical correlation
between the violent incidents and areas of deprivation. While gang violence
was cited as a major factor in the violence, Mr. Featherstone argued that
only a small number of rioters were members of gangs, and even then they
behaved in ways not typical of gang rivalries. Throughout his presentation,
Mr. Featherstone echoed a number of elements that had been noted previously by other speakers, specifically the importance of the social context,
the dynamics of groups, the emotional response to witnessing violence,
and the potential for epidemics to peak and then decline, in describing the
complexities of this event.

In discussing potential interventions to reduce violence related not just
to the riots, but the preexisting social and economic conditions, Mr. Featherstone noted the importance of empowering individuals to not identify
as victims or perpetrators. He also noted the importance of developing
community–law enforcement relationships to build trust. He stated, for
example, that in the case of Mark Duggan, some of the immediate incendi-
ary violence might have been prevented if police had spoken to the family
and conveyed a sense of working with the community. Speaker and planning committee member Charlotte Watts of the London School of Hygiene
and Tropical Medicine shared concerns that while interruption programs
reduced street violence, they did not address the underlying issues that

exacerbated the tense situation. Mr. Featherstone concurred, and noted that such reforms would take years to implement, while reducing retaliatory violence could be an easier issue to address in the short term.

The "Arab Spring" and Iraq

The "Arab Spring" is a term coined to describe events across the Middle East and North Africa (MENA) characterized by wide-scale populist uprisings against dictatorial governments. While many of the events are continuing, the uprisings have been likened to the "Autumn of Nations" that occurred in Eastern Europe in 1989. The singular event that was said to have begun the wave was the self-immolation of Tunisian Mohamed Bouazizi on December 18, 2010, as an act of protest against police and government corruption. Immediately in response, protests cropped up throughout Tunisia, and eventually led to the toppling of the government. A month later, similar protests swept through Egypt, and spread to Bahrain, Libya, Syria, and Yemen. Protests also occurred in Algeria, Iran, Iraq, Jordan, Morocco, and Oman and continued to spread through the region.

Unlike the UK riots, a contained trajectory of events has not presented itself in the MENA region. Additionally, many forms of violence have been reported, not limited to political conflict, but also spikes in interpersonal violence (e.g., sexual harassment). Ms. Al-Suwaij noted that as collective violence has destabilized communities, it has normalized the use of other types of violence, echoing comments by other speakers about different "syndromes" of violence.

Ms. Al-Suwaij also spoke of her experience with violence in Iraq, going back to her time as a student during Saddam Hussein's regime, and the protests that occurred then, reminiscent of those occurring now. She noted that much of the violence is sectarian or interethnic and she is exploring opportunities to reduce such violence. She established Ambassadors for Peace, a program she has sold with varying degrees of success to community and religious leaders in various locations in Iraq. In describing her experience, she noted that much of the conflict that occurs is related to simmering resentment, and is often set off by something innocuous, such as two children arguing over a soccer game. Thus her approach to mediating conflict draws heavily on the Cure Violence (formerly known as CeaseFire) model, and aims to interrupt retaliatory or tribal violence related to preexisting grievances. She noted that in one of three areas in Basrah, in which her program has been operating for 3 years, intertribal violence has been reduced to zero. She also discussed plans to scale up the program and move to other areas.

Ms. Al-Suwaij also noted challenges in the Ambassadors for Peace program, notably continuing political violence, lack of trust in law enforcement (an issue that is being addressed), and the inability to intervene as successfully in other forms of violence, such as domestic violence. She noted that it is still taboo to talk about domestic violence, and much of it is vastly underreported. When her interrupters hear about violence in families, they attempt to address it, but the existing legal structure prevents significant addressing of the issue. She also noted that, in peer group sessions of only women, some conversation around gender equality, gender norms, and violence against women is introduced.

INTERRUPTION AND APPLICATION

Panelists in the afternoon of the second day described some approaches to interruption, and challenges and opportunities to scale up. Before the panel, participants watched the documentary film *The Interrupters*, which chronicles the work of four violence interrupters as part of the CeaseFire Illinois initiative (CeaseFire Illinois is a Cure Violence program). CeaseFire Illinois, the program initially developed by speaker and planning committee member Gary Slutkin of the University of Illinois at Chicago, uses individuals called interrupters to halt the further spread of violence. These interrupters are respected in the community and usually have some history of violence themselves. They intervene when violence occurs, usually to prevent further spread or to prevent retaliation. They also work with high-risk individuals in the community to reduce tensions and other conditions that might result in violence.

In introducing the film, facilitator and planning committee member Brian Flynn of the Uniformed Services University School of Medicine explored some key concepts in the natural cycle of violence. He noted, referencing Stephen Pinker's book *The Better Angels of Our Nature*, that traditionally violence is lower in urban versus rural areas. Pinker's premise is that rule of law and governing systems are responsible for reducing violence, but in areas where violence spikes, people may not feel that rules apply to them, or systems are capable of upholding justice. Dr. Flynn also stated that, per Pinker, as women become more empowered, violence decreases as well. He urged the audience to consider these points as they watched the film. Finally, he posited that as previous discussions highlighted the observation of violence (either near or far) as a risk factor for future perpetration or victimization, perhaps the observation of violence interruption could further the spread of prevention as well.

Community-Based Intervention

Following the film, speaker and CeaseFire Illinois program director Tio Hardiman spoke about the experience of the interrupters, the program, and potential for scaling up. He gave four examples of recent events, which transpired within an hour, that required the intervention of the interrupters: (1) an incident involving a man who stole his girlfriend's pain medication, prompting threats and retaliation from her sons; (2) an incident involving two men in a territorial altercation that had expanded to involve several others; (3) two men arguing over a woman; and (4) two men involved in an altercation over the sale of drugs, which the interrupters did not mediate, though they did ensure that the situation would not result in violence. Mr. Hardiman went on to note that CeaseFire interrupters worked with 1,100 high-risk individuals and mediated 800 conflicts in 2011.

In Chicago, homicide is the leading cause of death for 15- to 24-year-olds, and Mr. Hardiman estimated that in the past decade, potentially 5,000 homicides have occurred. He described the circumstances in which many young individuals involved in violence and crime grow up with the mentality of needing to shoot first, to not be victimized, and to find ways to leave the structural poverty of family neighborhoods behind. He noted that violence is often normalized in these situations, and has lasting effects in a number of settings, such as schools, where children have difficulty learning because of fear of events outside of school. He noted that businesses often leave neighborhoods because of the destabilizing effect of violence. He also noted the importance of addressing issues on "the front end," that is, intercepting rumors of potential violence, and intervening before it occurs.

The Cure Violence model, in addition to interrupting the spread of violence, also aims to address social and group norms and behaviors around violence. Some of the work involves reaching out to individuals and assisting them with employment or education. In addition to the work of the interrupters, outreach workers are constantly in communities monitoring the pulse and providing educational opportunities. The interrupters also liaise with local law enforcement and mediate conflicts with victims of shootings who end up in hospitals.

School-Based Intervention

Speaker Patrick Burton of the Center for Justice and Crime Prevention in South Africa shared his experience with working in schools in South Africa to reduce violence in youth. The program, in particular, was interested in preventing "low-level," high-frequency violence such as bullying and dating violence, and in improving academic outcomes. He also noted the importance of addressing the social milieu and how students relate to one another in terms of forming more positive relationships. Dr. Burton spoke of data issues, particularly a lack of insightful, robust data, often due to non-reporting because of fear of the perception that schools are not safe. Despite this, he estimates that about 15 percent of students had experienced violence in the previous 12 months.

In describing the approach, Dr. Burton explained the "whole-school" approach, in which the program works with all stakeholders in school-based learning, including the teachers, students, parents, school governing body, and policy makers. It is also embedded in communities, working with families and homes in which students are experiencing or at risk of experiencing violence. The program places responsibility of identifying priorities and interventions on the schools, while providing guidance on response and prevention. Schools are shown how to identify safe and unsafe spaces within schools, how to manage and respond to reports of violence or threats of violence, and how to demonstrate action on such reports.

Dr. Burton went on to explore some of the challenges faced in the program and in scaling up. In 2005, the program was piloted in 85 schools; it is now active in just over 2,000 schools nationally. It is also currently being developed to other sites outside South Africa. Two formal outcome evaluations have been performed, and several informal process evaluations. He noted challenges in accountability, such as who is responsible for violence occurring and for response or lack thereof; ownership, management, and institutionalization. These challenges are especially difficult because effective school managers are often moved around. There are also challenges in supporting schools, whose primary task is education, to also work toward providing safe environments and the shared vision of what a safe school means—not just physical security.

The social context in South Africa has played a strong role in the exacerbation of violence, including a sizeable percentage of students (16 percent) having family members who have committed acts of violence and are currently incarcerated. Mr. Burton noted that the success of the school intervention program has been dependent on the integration with home-based efforts to address family violence. In the most successful sites, where there has been integration with parenting programs and the school's efforts, school-based violence has dropped significantly, some down to zero.

Family Violence Prevention and Interruption

In thinking about interrupting violence at the family level, speaker Valerie Maholmes of the *Eunice Kennedy Shriver* National Institute for Child Health & Human Development explored a series of studies being funded by her institute. She noted particularly how much of the research focuses on early development, and the importance of both the research and that age group in framing violence prevention. The first study she noted is that of Judith Langlois, which looks at the development of appearance-based stereotypes in children. Children naturally differentiate between more and less attractive appearances, but it is the observation of differential behavior by parents that ingrains value in appearance. Throughout life, these biases are more firmly established through repeated observation, and serve as barriers to receptivity of counterstereotypic messaging. Dr. Maholmes noted that the important implication here is that this work may prompt the development of interventions that ameliorate negative judgment based on attractiveness, and learning about these mechanisms may help inform evidence-based practice.

Dr. Maholmes went on to describe an intervention in India designed by Suneeta Krishnan, called DIL-MIL (Hindi: "hearts together"), which leverages the role of mothers-in-law to reduce violence against daughters-in-law. She noted that women are vulnerable to gender-based violence because they often have to acquiesce to the marital family, and that efforts to empower women must take into account social and family dynamics. She noted that mothers in law are crucial entry points, but people do not often realize that their role can be pivotal. This intervention brings these dyads together and, using social-cognitive theory, educates and empowers the women to reduce gender-based violence. Finally, Dr. Maholmes described a study by Amy Marshall looking at aggression within families, disaggregating interparental aggression (IPA) and parent-to-child aggression (PCA) to see if the two co-occur, if PCA is an outcome of IPA, if either or both have a "spillover" effect to violence between other family members (i.e., sibling-to-sibling) or outside the family.

In response to a question from a participant, Dr. Maholmes noted that intergenerational transmission of violence is strongly influenced by the normalization of violent behavior within families and the internalization of such by girls. She posited that useful interventions in breaking this cycle would need to include messaging around self-worth and self-esteem, as well as the ability to show other types of relationships.

Trauma-Informed Approaches

Speaker John Rich of the Drexel University School of Public Health spoke of the importance of the trauma-informed approach to violence prevention, noting that trauma is at the center of violence and that "hurt people hurt people." He also referenced other words from Sandra Bloom from the Drexel University School of Public Health about reframing inquiry from asking about what is wrong with someone to asking what happened to someone, knowing that early adversity and stress can have deleterious effects. In thinking about how to approach the interruption of violence in the health care setting, Dr. Rich noted the importance of examining these roots of trauma because patients who present with physical injury often have psychological injury as well. Failing to address those secondary injuries runs the risk of retraumatizing the individual. He also pointed out that the "injured" included not only the individual with the injury, but those who might have witnessed the violence, and potentially even those who work with the injured and traumatized; thus, understanding trauma across populations informs violence prevention at larger scales.

Dr. Rich also stated that violence is a recurrent disease, with high risks of recurrence. He cited some studies that show, 5 years out, that 45 percent of those with serious injury have experienced another serious injury, and 20 percent of them are dead. Of that 20 percent, 70 percent had substance abuse listed as a contributory cause. In other situations he referenced, young men who present with serious injury have high rates of posttraumatic stress disorder (PTSD), hypervigilance, and history of childhood adversity. Dr. Rich also pointed out that perpetrators are also at risk of PTSD symptoms, so it is not just victims.

Hospital-based interventions that are trauma-informed have been known to work. Shock Trauma in Baltimore has an intervention that has shown a reduction in involvement in the criminal justice system for its patients. Dr. Rich explained that hospital-based interventions are about recognizing the additional trauma faced, as a bigger picture approach to reducing violence. The interventions screen for past trauma and provide guidance in navigating systems, both medical and criminal justice, which might also potentially retraumatize. It also provides an outlet for aggression or rage, usually conversation with a case worker, as a means to reduce the potential for retaliatory violence. Finally, he noted it is important to include direct trauma recovery assistance as well, citing a few in use with evidence to back effectiveness.

Most salient though, Dr. Rich noted, is system-wide transformation into treating trauma as a cause and not just as an outcome, and to reflect on the comorbidity of different forms of violence, in the context of trauma. In addition, educating the community on trauma and its effects would provide a more nuanced perspective, including structural violence and intergenerational oppression. He noted especially that moving the conversation out of just hospitals and into a number of partnering organizations as well as the community would be the most effective approach.

Key Messages Raised by Individual Speakers

- The spread of violence has a number of complex factors, including social and contextual undercurrents that fuel frustration, anger, and mistrust in systems (Featherstone, Flynn, Rich).
- Finding a key leverage or entry point could optimize interventions (Hardiman, Maholmes).
- Recognizing and addressing the fundamentals of trauma provides a holistic approach to hospital- and community-based interventions (Hardiman, Rich).
- Scaling up requires attention to a number of factors, including accountability and finding and working with partners (Al-Suwaij, Burton, Hardiman).

Part II

Papers and Commentary
from Speakers

II.1

VIOLENCE: CONTAGION, GROUP MARGINALIZATION, AND RESILIENCE OR PROTECTIVE FACTORS

Carl C. Bell, M.D.
Community Mental Health Council, Inc.
Department of Psychiatry, College of Medicine,
University of Illinois at Chicago

The relationships among contagion, group marginalization, and resilience form a complex issue that does not lend itself to quantitative methodology, but rather is best studied using qualitative methods. Thus, having a historical perspective is an important attribute to understand appropriately the phenomenon of violence as it relates to contagion, group marginalization, and resilience or protective factors. Furthermore, in order to have a coherent discussion about violence, we must first understand which type of violence we are focusing on, as violence is a very complex and multi-determined phenomenon. In addition, we must understand the science.

The Need for Good Science

To understand this complex problem, we must understand the need for good science. Unfortunately, there is a fundamental scientific problem with understanding violence, whether it is directed toward others or self-directed. The reality is that these phenomena, while being the third or leading cause of death for some population groups, such as teens or young black males, respectively, are actually rare events. The reality is that suicide rates tend to be 11 suicides/100,000 (IOM, 2002) and homicide rates are about 9/100,000 (Douglas and Bell, 2011). Even if you focus on non-Hispanic black people who have rates of homicide of around 33/100,000 or gun homicides with rates of 58/100,000, these are low base rates and developing statistical power to differentiate between an experimental intervention and control is very difficult. Accordingly, the 2002 Institute of Medicine report *Reducing Suicide: A National Imperative* noted that to prove a suicide prevention intervention is evidence-based, a study would need 5 to 10 population studies with 100,000 persons per study to get enough statistical power to show that either a suicide or homicide prevention study works (IOM, 2002). Because the homicide rates are actually lower than the suicide rates, despite many scientific claims to the contrary, apparently one would need an equally large population to prove a homicide prevention intervention is evidence-based, and neither of these two studies has been done.

Types of Violence

Having formally studied the phenomenon of violence for more than 30 years, we proposed that there were many different forms of violence, which required different prevention, intervention, and postintervention strategies (Bell, 1997). As identified by Baker and Bell (1999), such types of violence include

- group or mob violence;
- individual violence;
- systemic violence, such as war, racism, and sexism;
- institutional violence, such as preventing inmates from getting the benefit of prophylactic medications to prevent hepatitis;
- hate-crime violence, such as terrorism;
- multicide (e.g., mass murder, murder sprees, and serial killing);
- psychopathic violence;
- predatory violence, also known as instrumental or secondary violence;
- interpersonal altercation violence, also known as expressive or primary violence (e.g., domestic violence, child abuse, elder abuse, and peer violence);
- drug-related violence, such as systemic drug-related violence (whereby drug dealers kill to sell drugs), pharmacological (whereby an individual perpetrates violence because of drug intoxication), economic-compulsive (whereby a drug addict uses violence to obtain drugs), and negligent (e.g., a drunk driver who kills a pedestrian);
- gang-related violence;
- violence by mentally ill individuals;
- lethal violence directed toward others (homicide);
- lethal violence directed toward self (suicide);
- violence by organically brain-damaged individuals;
- legitimate/illegitimate violence; and
- non lethal violence.

Observations About Types of Violence Regarding Issues of Contagion, Group Marginalization, and Resilience

Culture Destroys and Culture Protects

Culture destroys Black communities in Chicago experience discrimination, stigma, and injustice at higher rates than their white counterparts. Consider the science that illustrates white males perpetrate similar levels of violence as black males (HHS, 2001) and engage in more illegal drug use; however, the majority of children and young adults who are incarcerated for these offenses are people of color. There also have been well-known allegations that Chicago police forced confessions of murder from innocent black men, several of whom were on death row until DNA evidence proved their innocence. For example, police officer Jon Burge, fired after the Police Board determined he had used torture, was convicted on counts of obstruction of justice and perjury arising out of a civil suit in which Burge was named a participant in the abuse or torture of people in custody (Stein, 1993). Structurally, we understand that most mid- and large-size cities have more absolute numbers of low-income whites than low-income blacks, but there are few low-income white neighborhoods because low-income whites have scattered-site housing. Police have a more difficult time finding and incarcerating illegal drug users when they live in scattered-site housing. Therefore, blacks who use illegal drugs are incarcerated more often than whites who use illegal drugs; this is one of the reasons for the disproportionate percentage of incarcerated black people.

In Canada, children from First Nations communities were removed from their families and told their culture was not acceptable, resulting in individuals within First Nations communities losing their cultural protective factors, which ultimately led to many of them engaging in the risky behaviors of suicide and intragroup homicide. Within these communities, alcoholism is common. For every one child in Canadian juvenile detention centers without fetal alcohol syndrome, 19 children have fetal alcohol spectrum disorders (Popova et al., 2011). Bell (2012) has proposed that many disruptive behaviors leading to incarceration results from fetal alcohol exposure (FAE). It is well known that FAE is a leading cause of speech and language disorders, attention deficit hyperactivity disorder, and other developmental or cognitive disorders (IOM, 1996). These are often responsible for affect dysregulation, which leads to disruptive behaviors, which in turn leads to incarceration.

These phenomena increase marginalization, thus facilitating fertile ground for promoting the contagion of violence. A perfect example is the victimization of Rodney King by police that spread into the African American community and resulted in mob violence. Thus, when we talk about violence and the contagion of violence, we must also discuss the systemic violence of racism and imperialism that historically spread across the world.

Culture protects   While doing HIV prevention work in Durban, South Africa, it was striking that 40 percent of the Zulu people were HIV positive, 6 percent of the white South Africans were HIV positive, but only 1 percent of the Indian South Africans were HIV positive. The conclusion was that the Indian South African culture protected them, while the Zulu culture and its protective influence had been stripped from them, making them vulnerable to risky activities, such as risky sexual behavior, substance abuse, and violence. The white South African culture also is eroding, resulting in higher levels of HIV-positive individuals (Murray, 2012).

Contagion of Suicide and Mass Murder

In discussing self-directed violence, we understand the phenomena of contagion of suicide (Phillips et al., 1992) and how the mass media can cause what is referred to as cluster suicide, copycat suicide, and suicide contagion. Accordingly, in an effort to reduce this phenomenon of contagion, this recognition resulted in the "Reporting on Suicide: Recommendations for the Media."[1] Given that certain types of mass murders often lead to suicide (Petee et al., 1997), it is proposed that these mass murders are actually suicides preceded by mass murder (Bell and McBride, 2010a). One could hypothesize that when the media publicizes events such as the ones that occurred in Columbine High School; Platte Canyon High School; an Amish school in Nickel Mines, Pennsylvania; Virginia Tech; and Northern Illinois University, such "suicides preceded by mass murder" are inadvertently promoted. We understand the high level of public interest in sensational news stories; nevertheless, unless we understand that an individual suicide is the dynamic driving the mass murder behavior, we will continue to inadvertently encourage this behavior. The difficulty is that electronic media is so ubiquitous; it would be difficult to design a study as Phillips (1974) did when we only had to contend with local print media. We need a consensus meeting to discuss these issues and figure out how to responsibly report on "suicides preceded by mass murders," or the hypothesized contagion will likely continue.

Interpersonal Violence

Regarding the type of violence known as interpersonal violence, we understand this type is responsible for most violence. Furthermore, although different cultural, racial, and ethnic groups have different rates of different types of violence (e.g., Latinos have more gang-related violence), we understand that interpersonal violence is more common in the African American community; however, from the mid-1970s to the mid-1990s, African American domestic violence decreased from 16/100,000 to 3/100,000 (Greenfield et al., 1998). Why? Because the number of domestic violence shelters increased dramatically, reducing the number of battered African

---

[1] See http://www.sprc.org/sites/sprc.org/files/library/sreporting.pdf.

American women who turned to committing violence against their partner as a means to stop being battered.

Other Forms of Violence

One form of violence that has not been studied adequately is violence by organically brain-damaged individuals (Bell et al., 1985; Bell, 1986, 1987; Bell and Kelly, 1987). Although there is no evidence for the reason for this lack of study, it can be hypothesized that the major reason for this oversight is the marginalization of those afflicted with head injury that ultimately results in their explosive behavior. It is hoped the recent "discovery" of this problem in football players will reduce the marginalization of this population resulting in appropriate study of the issue yielding more prevention and treatment strategies. The issue of legitimate versus illegitimate violence is another issue we must explore.

Protective Factors That Cultivate Resilience
Against Various Types of Violence

Social Fabric Prevents Contagion of Violence

As director of the Institute of Juvenile Research, where child psychiatry began and where the issue of family and community violence was addressed more than 100 years ago, I am aware of a great deal of relevant history that pertains to contagion, group marginalization, and resilience or protective factors as they relate to violence. The lessons learned from this history are quite instructive to this discussion. In Chicago in 1871, the Great Fire created a lot of instability in a city with a population that was 70 percent either foreign-born or first-generation. The results were families who, due to being disrupted by poverty and unfamiliar community circumstances as result of immigration, were unable to provide stable family environments and to flourish. Evidence of this problem was the extraordinarily high rate of European immigrant domestic violence in Chicago from 1875 to 1920 (Adler, 2003). Seeing the problem, Jane Addams made efforts to found Hull House "to aid in the solution of the social and industrial problems which are engendered by the modern conditions of life in a great city." In 1889, Addams and her colleagues established a Juvenile Court in Illinois to distinguish between delinquency and criminality. The procedures of this new institution were not to be adversarial; rather it was "primarily protective and educational rather than punitive, and the commission of a child to a correctional institution is deemed to be for his welfare and not for the sole purpose of inflicting penalty." Ten years later, in 1909, these foresighted women convinced the state of Illinois to discover the cause of delinquency;

the Juvenile Psychopathic Institute (later called the Institute for Juvenile Research, or IJR) was created, and neurologist William Healy was hired to be the first director. Later, IJR researchers Shaw and McKay (1942) noted delinquency was less due to biological, ethnic, or cultural factors and more due to social disruption eroding formal and informal social control in specific transitional neighborhoods (delinquency areas) in a city.

Fifty years ago, the science was not as advanced as it is now. The research designs were empirical and qualitative instead of being quantitative, and much of the IJR's research was mostly biographical. Thus, the statistical methodology was very primitive by today's standards and multivariate influences could not be studied well enough statistically. However, despite this lack of scientific methodology, it is interesting that the IJR's observations were correct. Their observations were that children's biology was not causing delinquency, but rather it was the lack of social fabric in the new immigrant communities. Of course, this finding predated by 50 years the seminal research of Sampson et al. (1997) that coined the term "collective efficacy."

Another example of how protective factors cultivate resiliency, which in turn is protective against contagion of violence, specifically cluster or copycat suicide, is found in building protective factors around vulnerable populations of potentially suicidal individuals. Because 20,000/100,000 people in the United States suffer from depression, 5,000/100,000 attempt suicide, and 11/100,000 actually complete suicide, something must be protecting people (Health Care Innovations Exchange Team, 2012). Accordingly, because youth engage in multiple risky behaviors due to their immature brain development, we have likened adolescents to be like cars with just gasoline, but no brakes and steering wheels, that is, community or social fabric (Bell and McBride, 2010b). These protective factors can be cultivated (Bell, 2001) and have been proposed as a strategy of suicide prevention. A specific example of infusing protective factors to prevent suicide occurs when, in an effort to prevent copycat or cluster suicide after a successful suicide, the victim's friends are screened for suicidality and then provided with preventive services (Brent et al., 1989).

Research has indicated that children who are sexually and physically abused are more likely to engage in suicidal behavior compared to children who are not abused (IOM, 2002). However, children with protective factors in their lives have fewer traumatic stress drivers of suicidal and other-directed violent behavior than children without these protective factors (Griffin et al., 2011). Thus, it is possible to cultivate resiliency in these populations as well.

Finally, based on years of public health research and work, the Seven Field Principles for Health Behavior Change are appropriate universal guiding principles to infuse protective factors in populations at risk for various types of violence: (1) rebuilding the village; (2) access to modern and ancient technology; (3) connectedness; (4) building self-esteem (a sense of power, uniqueness, connectedness, and models); (5) cultivating social and emotional skills; (6) reestablishing the adult protective shield; and (7) minimizing trauma. These efforts have led to the maxim that "risk factors are not predictive factors due to protective factors" (Bell et al., 2008).

II.2

SCHOOL-BASED VIOLENCE AND INTERRUPTION

Patrick Burton, Ph.D.
Center for Justice and Crime Prevention, South Africa

Introduction

Crime is one of the most significant challenges facing democratic South Africa, and young people between the ages of 12 and 21 are often at the receiving end of this escalating violence. Figures show that young people experience violence at rates that are exponentially higher than their adult counterparts (Leoschut and Burton, 2006). Given that this age cohort constitutes a significant proportion of the general population of South Africa, any efforts to reduce and prevent violence should incorporate components addressing child and youth violence. Furthermore, substantial evidence shows that violence and victimization against young people is closely correlated to later violence; any attempt to adequately address violence at a community or societal level must therefore take into account the levels and nature of violence experienced by young people and children.[2]

Schools in South Africa are consistently shown to be one of the most common sites of violence perpetrated against children and youth. This is not surprising because children spend most of their time away from home in the school environment. In 2005, the first National Youth Victimization Study in South Africa revealed that 11.5 percent of youth between ages 12 and 22 feel anxious and fearful while at school. These feelings of apprehension were most frequently attributed to the fear of criminals (52.5 percent), of being harmed (21.4 percent), of classmates (18.3 percent), and of educators (4.8 percent). Fear was not limited to the school environment, but was

---

[2] See, for example, Farrington, D., and P. Welsh. 2007. *Saving children from a life of crime.* Oxford University Press, Oxford; Haggerty, R., et al. 1996. *Stress, risk, and resilience in children and adolescents: Processes, mechanisms and interventions.* Cambridge: Cambridge University Press; and Cornell, D. G., and M. J. Mayer. 2010. Why do school order and safety matter? *Educational Researcher* (39)1:7-15.

also often associated with the journey to and from school, as reported by 16.8 percent of the more than 4,000 young persons surveyed.

Being raised in violent social contexts influences children's understanding of how the social world works (CIET Africa, 2004). In addition to undermining their sense of safety and security, creating feelings of fear and anxiety, disrupting eating and sleeping patterns, and leading to difficulties concentrating at school, direct and indirect exposure to violence can result in the adoption of violence as a legitimate means of resolving conflicts and as a way of protecting oneself from harm (Boxford, 2006). All of these factors make it extremely difficult, if not impossible, for quality learning to occur and have thus been found to contribute to grade repetition and the non-completion of schooling. This suggests that the vast majority of children and youth in South Africa are deprived of their right to live and learn in a safe environment that is free of violence or its threat.

This paper will provide insights into just one approach to addressing school violence in South Africa, and into some of the lessons learned as the program has evolved and adapted based on several evaluations. The program is the Hlayiseka School Safety Toolkit, and forms the basis for the National Department of Basic Education's developing school safety framework.

The Approach

The departure point for the toolkit recognizes that violence has physical, social, psychological, and environmental roots, and that, to end it, we need to address it at multiple levels and from different sectors of society. The complex and dynamic interactions of all the environments (e.g., communities, homes) in which young people live out their life are what impact the experience and nature of violence, within the school environment in particular.

Another point needs to be emphasized at the outset. While the most common reaction to the phrase "school-based violence" may lead the mind to jump to high-profile incidents of school shootings, or increasingly maybe highly reported cases of cyberbullying, for example, these are not the manifestation of violence within the learning environment that we should be most concerned. Rather, these are isolated, high-profile, and sensationalized incidents, and while tragic, are not where the problem lies. Rather, the real problem lies in the apparently minor, but repetitive, acts of violence. These acts lead to the most frequent negative consequences of violence in schools: dropping out, truancy, school (and often social) phobia, depression, and lack of self-confidence in students. These acts can also negatively affect educational outcomes and attachment to schools and learning, which we know are among some of the most significant protective factors for young people (Debarbiaux, 2003).

The Hlayiseka Toolkit uses a training methodology built on the principle of a "whole school approach" to school safety. This approach posits that the responsibility for and successful approach to school safety requires the commitment of all those who constitute the schooling environment: learners, educators, principals, parents, and the school governance structures. It also advocates that a safe school needs to be first and foremost a functional school. In short, the more effectively and democratically a school is managed, generally, the higher the likelihood of a positive impact on safety outcomes (Gottfredson, 2001). The approach provides the basis for the South African School Safety Policy that is being developed; details the implementation of standardized school policies regarding learner and educator conduct, rights, responsibilities, and expectations; and requires buy-in from principals, learners, educators, school safety teams, and school governing bodies.

The toolkit acknowledges that each school is at a different point in its journey toward school safety and that available resources and capacity differ from school to school. The toolkit thus allows for the least resourced school to find an appropriate entry point into the system as well as the most-resourced school. The toolkit is built on a foundation composed of four building blocks: Be prepared to prevent and manage problems and violence; be aware of what is happening at school; take action when something happens; and finally, take steps to build a caring school. Each building block assists the school to work systematically toward achieving school safety. The broad objectives of the toolkit are to help the school to understand and identify security issues and threats; guide schools to respond effectively to security issues and threats; establish reporting systems and manage reported incidents appropriately; monitor the school's progress over time; and integrate existing departmental policy and legislation to ensure that school safety is not an "add on." On a purely programmatic level, the whole-school approach provides each school with the tools to themselves understand and identify threats to safety; respond effectively to violence and threats of violence (including early identification of threats); and prevent, report, and manage threats and incidents effectively. These effectively constitute a process of diagnosing, planning, acting, and monitoring. Most importantly, such an approach is designed to improve school management rather than the range of additional activities and interventions that may be offered. It does not serve to replace, for example, life skills, conflict mediation, positive discipline, or after-school care activities that may be implemented at the school level.

Implementation and Lessons

Although the implementation of the toolkit in some instances resulted
in decreases in school incidents by up to 23 percent (when controlled for
external variables), there were also sufficient examples of a whole-school
approach failing to adequately address violence issues in schools to warrant
further exploration into what works and what does not, particularly as
within South Africa, where the approach was to be scaled up from the original 85 pilot sites to more than 2,200 schools nationally. This assessment of
what was impacting the success and failure of the toolkit has increasingly
been done through the application of a public health lens, together with
a greater recognition placed on the interactions among different environments in which, on individual and community levels, learners and educators live, and on an institutional level, the school is situated. This reflects
findings into the efficacy of school-specific interventions to reduce violence,
which show that comprehensive school-based interventions achieve greater
and more sustained impact than single interventions.[3]

The approach thus requires that the school-based intervention is embedded in what is happening in the homes of children, and the communities in
which the school is situated. This reflects the findings of the report on school
violence released by the Special Representative of the Secretary-General on
Violence Against Children, which argues that community outreach (i.e.,
engaging with parents and community members) is a prerequisite for establishing safe schools. Accordingly, a revised model of Hlayiseka was piloted
in a number of sites in urban environments throughout South Africa, and
paired with different family and community-based interventions, determined through a process of site-based safety auditing. Three particular
family-based interventions were prioritized in the different sites: healthy
masculinities for fathers, and young fathers in particular; family role modeling; and parenting interventions. These were introduced in a phased
manner, and resulted in further reductions of up to 18 percent in levels of
violence within each of the targeted schools. Other indirect impact was reported by school principals, primarily in the form of improved educational
performance in class tests and examinations. However, the degree to which
the improved impact is a direct measure of the additional family-directed
interventions, or the effect of a longer implementation period of the toolkit
at each school, has not been measured.

---

[3] See, for example, Farrington, D., and B. Welsh. 2007. *Saving children from a life of crime.*
Oxford, UK: Oxford University Press; and Swearer, S. M., K. S. Bevin, D. L. Espelage, W. L.
Kingsbury, J. Peugh, and A. B. Siebecker. 2006. A socioecological model for bullying preven-
tion and intervention in early adolescence: An exploratory examination. In S. R. Jumerson
and M. J. Furlong, Eds., *Handbook of school violence and school safety.* Mahwah, NJ: Lawrence
Erlbaum Associates.

Challenges

A number of challenges have been documented through the evaluation process that impact the potential of the toolkit to successfully interrupt violence at and relating to the school. These arise particularly from the need to embed the interaction and intervention in the broader environments:

1. The consecutive addressing of protective factors outside the control of the school, and parents or caregivers. The greatest impact is seen when interventions specifically targeting school safety occur concurrently with tailored family and community interventions.
2. Ownership is key, particularly in environments where effective and efficient school managers are scarce. The most effective usually serve as project champion and are usually also those who are moved on in relatively quick succession to where the need for effective leadership is seen as greatest. This often leaves an ownership vacuum, with particular approaches or interventions seen as being the property of an individual; hence there is no institutionalization of the approach.
3. Accountability from the school level up to districts, provinces, and national levels. Most often, accountability, where it exists at all, stops at a district or provincial level. School principals are often faced with the same challenge as police station commanders— whereas increased reports of violence may initially signal an increase in reporting and trust and action, rather than an actual increase in the levels of crime. Furthermore, competition among districts and provinces results in data not being fed up the chain to national levels, which results in an inaccurate picture, if any picture at all.
4. Furthermore, an ongoing debate as to the core business of the school, and the Department of Basic Education, which sees learning as its core business, rather than enhancing the safety of the school. Safety is perceived by many to still be a police or parental function.
5. Not unrelated to this is the blame-laying game, where educators shift the blame for violent behavior to parents, and vice versa— often resulting in a lack of engagement between the two and a lack of willingness to engage.

II.3

CONTAGION OF COLLECTIVE VIOLENCE: CONTAGION
FROM ETHNOPOLITICAL VIOLENCE TO OTHER
FORMS OF AGGRESSION AND VIOLENCE[4]

Eric F. Dubow, Ph.D.
The University of Michigan and Bowling Green State University

Wars, ethnopolitical violence, and state-perpetrated violence are prevalent throughout the world, and a risk for such violence exists in many countries. The Economist Intelligence Unit (2009) calculates a Political Instability Index based on four factors that predict outbreaks of social and political unrest: higher infant mortality rates; extreme cases of economic or political discrimination against minorities; living in "a bad neighborhood" (if a country has at least four neighboring countries that suffered violent conflicts); and oppressive regime type. Once political instability results in violence, however, the consequences for children in the affected countries become even worse as violence begets more violence. In this paper, I focus on how exposure to ethnopolitical violence infects the community, the family, and the individual child with violence. I also describe evidence about some specific psychological processes accounting for how observed war violence leads the child to become more aggressive and violent.

The general idea of contagion of violence across levels of the social ecosystem is based on Bronfenbrenner's (1979, 2005) model of hierarchically nested ecosystems: ethnopolitical violence might produce direct or indirect effects on the child. The indirect effects occur in part because violence at the political/governmental level of the social ecology, what Bronfenbrenner described as the exosystem, infects violence at levels more proximal to the child (the microsystem)—the community, the school, and the family, which in turn have direct effects on the child.

War Affects Community-Level Indicators of Violence

Significant evidence shows that war affects community-level indicators of violence. Archer and Gartner (1976, 1984) reviewed studies showing that wars were related to subsequent postwar crimes in the community. The authors examined homicide rates in combatant and noncombatant comparison nations in World Wars I and II—homicide rates 5 years before and 5 years after war. In combatant nations, homicide rates increased in 19

---

[4] This research was supported by a grant from the *Eunice Kennedy Shriver* National Institute of Child Health & Human Development (Grant No. HD047814; L. Rowell Huesmann, Principal Investigator).

countries and decreased in 6; in noncombatant control countries, 7 countries decreased and 5 increased in homicide rates. Archer and Gartner noted that previous research in this area attributed effects of war on subsequent community-level crime to factors such as loosening of family ties and weakened respect for law, human life, and property. The authors examined several factors that could account for war effects on subsequent homicides, including whether the country won or lost the war and subsequent economic effects, and none of these factors accounted for the significant effects. Archer and Gartner argued that the effects were likely due to a legitimation hypothesis that stipulates that sanctioning of killing interculturally during times of war normalizes and legitimizes killing and other acts of violence intraculturally.

Landau found that during a 15-year period (1967-1982) in Israel, a monthly increase in security-related casualties predicted the number of homicides (Landau and Pfeffermann, 1988; Landau, 1997, 2003). This relation extended 1-5 months ahead. Landau also examined crime statistics comparing 2000 and 2001 (the year before and the year after the onset of Second Intifada): homicide rates increased 28 percent, robbery 11 percent, and road accident fatalities 16 percent. Landau and Pfeffermann (1988, p. 500) concluded, "Violence resulting from conflicts with out-groups (enemies) is generalized also toward in-group members in society. In other words, there is a gradual, consistent, and continuous process of erosion of basic social norms regarding violence in society."

As another example of war violence affecting a community-level indicator of violence, Miguel et al. (2008) examined the on-field behavior of European soccer players with different degrees of exposure to civil war in their home countries. The authors found a significant positive relationship between the number of years of civil war in a player's home country and his subsequent earning of yellow cards for aggressive behavior on the soccer field. The relationship was significant even when controlling for player positions, income, age, and league and team fixed effects.

War Affects Family-Level Indicators of Violence

Researchers also have reported that war violence and family-level violence co-occur. Landau (2003) found that during the First Intifada, there was a significant increase in domestic homicides in Israel. Similarly, Clark et al. (2010) found that in a Palestinian sample, married women's reports of their husbands' exposure to ethnopolitical violence was associated with acts of domestic violence. Catani et al. (2008, 2009) surveyed 287 Afghan and 286 Sri Lankan youths between the ages of 9 and 15. More than half witnessed three or more family violence events (e.g., interparental, parent-to-child, sibling-to-sibling); in both samples, a history of war trauma predicted domestic violence.

War Affects the Child's Aggressive Behavior

A fair amount of literature has been published recently on the damaging psychosocial effects of war on youth in Iraq, Palestine, Israel, Bosnia, Rwanda, Sierra Leone, Uganda, and Northern Ireland. Studies most commonly focus on posttraumatic stress. Only 12 of 95 studies of adolescents exposed to war violence published between 1972 and 2006 examined effects on problem behavior, Barber (2009) reported. Researchers in the Gaza Community Mental Health Programme (Qouta and El Sarraj, 1992; Qouta et al., 2008) reported that 38 percent of children during the First Intifada in Gaza developed aggressive behavior. In two samples of 12- to 16-year-olds, one during a peaceful time and one during the Second Intifada, witnessing and being victimized by war violence predicted children's self- and parent-reported aggression. In our own 3-year longitudinal study of 1,501 Israeli and Palestinian 8-, 11-, and 14-year-olds (Dubow et al., 2010; Landau et al., 2010; Boxer et al., 2012), exposure to ethnopolitical conflict/violence was related both to aggression and posttraumatic stress symptoms, even after controlling for a range of demographic and contextual factors. Political violence exposure predicted increases in violence at more proximal levels of the social ecology (e.g., school, community), but only political violence predicted subsequent aggression at peers across all three age groups.

A body of literature is also emerging on outcomes for child soldiers. Much of the research examines child soldiers in Sierra Leone and Uganda once they become reintegrated into their communities. In Sierra Leone, Betancourt et al. (2010) found that youth who wounded or killed others or survived rape reported more hostility and fighting with peers when they returned home. However, most of the associations between war exposure and subsequent outcomes were no longer significant once postconflict experiences were included in statistical models. Specifically, that study and other studies in Sierra Leone and Uganda (Annan et al., 2006; Klasen et al., 2010) showed that exposure to domestic violence, community violence, and the stigma of having been a child soldier—even though these youth were generally abducted into the armed warfare—predicted further problem behaviors. Family and community acceptance upon reintegration, literacy, and economic opportunities helped shape resilient outcomes.

Psychological Processes Accounting for the Contagion of War Violence to Individual Violence

Empirical research has identified a few psychological processes that appear to promote the contagion of violence. First, consistent with the legitimation-habituation hypothesis, exposure to violence seems to promote social cognitions that support and justify aggression (Huesmann and Kirwil, 2007). Observing violence promotes an aggressive way of thinking that includes fantasizing about aggression, normative beliefs that aggression is a justified response to solving social conflicts, and internalized scripts (guidelines for social behavior) for how to behave aggressively in social conflict situations. In our study of Israeli and Palestinian youth (Dubow et al., 2011), exposure to political violence led to increased aggressive fantasizing and increased normative beliefs that aggression is a justified way to solve interpersonal conflicts; in turn, these social cognitions affected subsequent aggressive behavior toward in-group peers.

In addition, Cummings et al. (2010, 2011) hypothesize that protection, safety, and security are core concerns in regulating emotions, cognitions, and behavior. In a 3-year longitudinal study of 10- to 17-year-olds in Northern Ireland, the authors found that sectarian violence affected problems at the family level (i.e., more marital conflict and less monitoring of the child, and child's emotional insecurity about living in the community), which in turn predicted the child's conduct problems and attention deficit-hyperactivity symptoms.

Conclusions

War and ethnopolitical violence are contagious: exposure to it stimulates violent behavior both in those who are victimized by it and in those who observe it. Studies support the idea of ethnopolitical violence as a higher level stressor or "legitimizer," increasing other forms of violence at lower levels of the social ecology, that is, within the community, within the schools, and within the family—with effects accruing on children's aggression. Psychological processes that account for this contagion of violence include the development of social cognitions that justify aggression and disruptions in children's emotional security about the community, as well as more general emotional dysregulation.

In terms of interventions for war-affected youth, Miller and Rasmussen (2010) suggested moving beyond the "trauma-focused model," which views war exposure as the critical intervention target. Instead, these authors advocated for a "psychosocial model," where the focus includes other critical ecological factors affecting development of youth in settings of persistent ethnopolitical conflict. Based on the contagion of violence across ecological levels, interventions may include school-based (e.g., violence prevention), community-based (e.g., neighborhood watch programs), and family-level (e.g., addressing spousal conflict) approaches. In addition, some have proposed approaches to preventing collective violence in the first place (Krug et al., 2002; De Jong, 2010) through international efforts to reduce poverty and inequality among groups in society; promote respect for human rights; adopt treaties restricting the use of landmines; decrease the production of biological, chemical, and nuclear weapons; and support accountable, democratic forms of government.

II.4

THE CONTAGION OF SUICIDAL BEHAVIOR

Madelyn S. Gould, Ph.D., M.P.H.
Columbia University and New York State Psychiatric Institute
and
Alison M. Lake, M.A.
New York State Psychiatric Institute

Introduction

Evidence has accumulated to support the idea that suicidal behavior is "contagious" in that it can be transmitted, directly or indirectly, from one person to another (Gould, 1990). This evidence is derived from three bodies of research: studies of the impact of media reporting on suicide, studies of suicide clusters, and studies of the impact on adolescents of exposure to a suicidal peer. In each case, suicide contagion can be viewed within the larger context of behavioral contagion or social learning theory. While research has also addressed the distinct but related topic of the contagion of nonsuicidal self-injurious behavior (Jacobson and Gould, 2009; Hawton et al., 2010; Whitlock, 2010), the current review focuses specifically on attempted and completed suicide.

Impact of Media Reporting on Suicide

Research into the impact of media stories about suicide has demonstrated an increase in suicide rates after both nonfictional and fictional stories about suicide. Most research in this area has addressed nonfictional reporting, which has been shown to have a more powerful effect (Stack, 2003). More than 50 studies on nonfictional stories reported in newspapers, on television, and more recently on the Internet, have yielded consistent findings. Suicide rates go up following an increase in the frequency of stories about suicide (e.g., Hagihara et al., 2007). Moreover, suicide rates go down following a decrease in the frequency of stories about suicide (e.g., Motto, 1970). A dose-response relationship between the quantity of reporting on completed suicide and subsequent suicide rates has consistently been demonstrated (e.g., Phillips, 1974; Phillips and Carstensen, 1986; Pirkis et al., 2006). Changes in suicide rates following media reports are more pronounced in regions where a higher proportion of the population is exposed (Etzersdorfer et al., 2004). The prevalence of Internet users, with access to Internet stories about suicide, has been associated with general population suicide rates in males, but not females (Hagihara et al., 2007; Shah, 2010).

The way suicide is reported is a significant factor in media-related suicide contagion, with more dramatic headlines and more prominently placed (i.e., front page) stories associated with greater increases in subsequent suicide rates (Phillips, 1974, 1979; Kuess and Hatzinger, 1986; Michel et al., 1995). Repetitive reporting on the same suicide and definitive labeling of the death as a suicide have also been associated with greater increases in subsequent suicide rates (Niederkrotenthaler et al., 2009, 2010). Content analyses of suicide newspaper reports from six countries with different suicide rates (Austria, Finland, Germany, Hungary, Japan, and the United States) found that attitudes toward suicide in newspaper reports varied by country, and that national suicide rates were higher in countries where media attitudes toward suicide were more accepting (Hungary) and suicide completers were more positively portrayed (Japan) (Fekete et al., 2001). Conversely, national suicide rates were lower in countries (Finland, Germany, and the United States) where reporting tended to portray the suicide victim and act of suicide in terms of psychopathology and abnormality, and to describe the negative consequences of the suicide. Moreover, media stories about individuals with suicidal ideation who used adaptive coping strategies to handle adverse events and did not attempt suicide have been negatively associated with subsequent suicide rates (Niederkrotenthaler et al., 2010).

The impact of media reporting on subsequent suicides is not monolithic, but interacts with characteristics of the reported suicide and characteristics of the media audience, as well as with characteristics of the media portrayal, as noted above. For example, celebrity suicides are more likely and the suicides of criminals are less likely to be followed by increased suicide rates (Stack, 2003; Niederkrotenthaler et al., 2009); individuals with a recent history of suicide attempt and/or a concurrent severe depression are more likely to attempt suicide in the wake of a media report (Cheng et al., 2007a,b).

Ecological studies of the impact of media on suicide rates, like those described above, meet four of Hill's five criteria for demonstrating causality (namely, consistency, temporality, strength of association, and coherence), but provide less convincing evidence of specificity (Hill, 1965; Gould, 1990; Insel and Gould, 2008). A handful of extant individual-level studies, however, have examined whether individuals who attempted suicide following a media story were exposed to and influenced by the media report, and have contributed evidence to support the specificity of the media effect. Hawton and colleagues (1999) conducted a study in emergency departments in the United Kingdom, examining the pattern of suicide attempts before and after a fictional Royal Air Force pilot took an overdose of paracetamol (i.e., acetaminophen) in an episode of a popular weekly TV drama. Presentations for self-poisoning increased by 17 percent in the week after the broadcast and 9 percent in the second week. Increases in overdoses using the specific drug used by the model were more marked than increases in other types of overdoses. The most compelling evidence of modeling from this study was that use of the specific drug for overdose among overdose patients who were viewers of the drama doubled after the episode in question, compared with overdose patients who were viewers of the drama prior to that episode. Twenty percent of the interviewed patients reported that the model had influenced their behavior. In a more recent study, 63 individuals who attempted suicide in Taipei, Taiwan, following the suicide of a young female pop singer were assessed for exposure to media reporting about her death. Forty-three (68 percent) respondents had been exposed to the media reporting, of whom 37 percent reported that the media stories influenced their suicide attempts (Chen et al., 2010). This study also demonstrated a positive modeling effect on the chosen method of suicide (burning charcoal inside a closed car), with an adjusted odds ratio of 7:3 (for additional evidence of a modeling effect based on choice of suicide method, see also Etzersdorfer et al., 2004; Cheng et al., 2007b; Chen et al., 2012).

Suicide Clusters

A suicide cluster is an excessive number of suicides occurring in close temporal and/or geographical proximity (Gould et al., 1989). Clusters occur primarily among teenagers and young adults, with between 1 percent and 5 percent of teen suicides occurring in clusters (Gould, 1990; Gould et al., 1990; Hazell, 1993). A case-control study of two teen suicide clusters in Texas indicated that the clusters included teens who had close personal relationships with others in the cluster, as well as teens from the same community who were not directly acquainted with one another (Davidson et al., 1989). When compared with matched living controls, suicide completers were more likely to have preexisting vulnerabilities (e.g., emotional illness, substance abuse problems, frequent changes of residence, recent or anticipated relationship break-up) that may have increased their susceptibility to suicide contagion.

It has been suggested that teen suicide clusters may result from the combination of assortative relating, the tendency for similar individuals (in this case, teens at high risk of suicide) to preferentially associate with one another, with shared life stress (Joiner, 2003). According to this argument, which should apply only to those teens within a suicide cluster who were directly acquainted with one another, teen suicides may cluster within a peer group because of high levels of preexisting vulnerability across the peer group, not because of suicide contagion. A recent study used agent-based computer simulation modeling to test this hypothesis and to explore the possible mechanisms behind suicide clustering (Mesoudi, 2009). As programmed in the simulation model, social learning was sufficient to generate suicide clusters localized both in time and space. The simulation model further found that assortative relating, also known as homophily, was likely to generate spatially localized suicide clusters among high-risk peer groups, but less likely to generate spatiotemporal suicide clusters and unlikely to generate purely temporal clustering of suicides. As the study's author notes, homophily seems to provide no reason why suicides should be clustered in time. Finally, the model confirmed that media effects, in combination with the effects of prestige and similarity biases, were capable of generating suicide clusters localized in time, but not space.

Even within spatiotemporal suicide clusters, where decedents are more likely to have direct contact with one another, media reporting on suicide can play a role. A recent analysis of the Foxconn suicides in China found support for a temporal clustering effect (Cheng et al., 2011). National (but not local) newspaper reporting on the suicides and the occurrence of a Foxconn suicide or suicide attempt were each associated with elevated chances of a subsequent suicide 3 days later, demonstrating the impact of both media-related contagion and direct contagion within the Foxconn company.

Impact on Adolescents of Exposure to a Suicidal Peer

Of 16 studies reviewed by Insel and Gould (2008) on the impact on adolescents of exposure to a suicidal peer, the majority found a significant association between exposure to the suicidal behavior of an adolescent peer and a subsequent adolescent suicide attempt. Odds ratios ranged from 2.8 to 11.0 for attempted suicide. Analysis of data on a nationally representative sample of U.S. high school students from the National Longitudinal Study of Adolescent Health (ADD Health) found that "teens who know friends or family members who have attempted suicide are about three times more likely to attempt suicide than are teens who do not know someone who attempted suicide" (Cutler et al., 2001). Girls were more likely to attempt suicide if they knew someone who had survived a suicide attempt, while boys were more likely to attempt suicide if they knew someone who had died by suicide. Teens who had not made a suicide attempt in wave one of the study were more likely to have attempted suicide in wave two if they knew someone who had attempted suicide in the interim; this temporal sequencing lends support for the role of contagion alongside the possible effect of assortative relationships among high-risk teens. In the context of exposure to the suicidal behavior of an intimate, contagion may operate via the impact on a vulnerable teen of stress or grief at the loss of a loved one, as well as via social learning about suicide.

Strategies to Prevent Suicide Contagion

A number of evidence-based interventions capable of combating suicide contagion have been developed. Studies have shown that it is possible to intervene to mitigate media-driven suicide contagion by implementing media guidelines for suicide reporting (Gould, 2001; Pirkis and Nordentoft, 2011). Media guidelines can interrupt the transmission of suicidality by identifying the types of media reporting through which suicidality is likely to be transmitted, and by modifying the volume and content of media reporting, with resultant decreases in suicide rates. For example, suicides in the Vienna subway system decreased by approximately 75 percent in 1987 following implementation of media guidelines for reporting on subway system suicides (Etzersdorfer et al., 1992). Applying media guidelines to new electronic media, including social networking websites, presents a new challenge to the suicide prevention community (Pirkis and Nordentoft, 2011; Robertson et al., 2012).

Screening for suicide risk can also interrupt the transmission of suicidality by identifying in advance individuals who may be susceptible to suicide contagion (Gould et al., 2009). In addition, suicide screening works to alleviate that susceptibility by enabling services to be directed to at-risk individuals identified by the screen. Key settings for suicide screening include schools and primary care practices. A range of school- and community-based psychosocial programs may also work to alleviate susceptibility to suicide contagion by, for example, changing adolescent peer norms through positive messaging (Wyman et al., 2010), or educating and empowering parents to communicate with teens (Toumbourou and Gregg, 2002). Finally, research suggests that coordinated postvention/crisis intervention efforts following a death by suicide may minimize and contain the effects of suicide contagion (Poijula et al., 2001; Hacker et al., 2008).

Conclusion

While the complex etiology of suicidal behavior is recognized (Gould et al., 2003), it has become increasingly apparent that suicide contagion exists and contributes to suicide risk along with psychopathology, biological vulnerability, family characteristics, and stressful life events. Strategies to prevent suicide contagion are essential and require ongoing evaluation.

II.5

THE POTENTIAL ROLE OF MIRROR NEURONS IN THE CONTAGION OF VIOLENCE

Marco Iacoboni, M.D., Ph.D.
David Geffen School of Medicine at
University of California, Los Angeles

Introduction

The social sciences have documented the contagion of violence with carefully controlled studies, including longitudinal studies over long periods of time. Indeed, some have proposed for the contagion of violence a model that mimics the spreading of infectious diseases (for both these issues, see other contributors to this workshop summary). This model captures well the phenomenon of contagion associated with violent behavior. The model, however, does not provide a biological mechanism that can plausibly account for the spreading of the behavior. Infectious diseases such as the flu have well-defined and well-studied causes, that is, the viruses that spread the flu from individual to individual. The missing link between the compelling social science studies on contagion of violence and the model of such contagion as an infectious disease is a biologically grounded mechanism. A recent neuroscience discovery, a type of brain cell called mirror neuron, may provide such a missing link. This paper summarizes what we know and do not know yet about mirror neurons and discusses the empirical findings from the neuroscience labs in light of potential implications for policy regarding the contagion of violence and its control.

Mirror Neurons: Original Findings

Mirror neurons were reported for the first time in the scientific literature exactly 20 years ago (Dipellegrino et al., 1992). The scientists who discovered mirror neurons were investigating a region of the monkey brain that controls actions with the hand (e.g., grasping an object, holding it, manipulating it, and so on), and actions with the mouth (e.g., as ingestive actions like biting and drinking, but also facial gestures like lip smacking, a social communication gesture of positive valence in monkeys) (Gentilucci et al., 1988; Rizzolatti et al., 1988). All of these actions are essential for normal everyday functioning. The scientists were studying the responses of the neurons, while the monkeys were performing those actions, to better understand how the brain controls motor behavior. Unexpectedly, the scientists found that some of the neurons were activated not only when the monkey was performing the action, but also when the monkey was simply observing somebody else making the same action. For instance, some grasping neurons activate when the monkey grasps a tiny object like a raisin (this type of grasp is called precision grip and is performed with the thumb and the index finger), but do not activate when the monkey grasps a large object like a banana (this type of grasp is called whole-hand prehension and requires the use of all fingers and the palm, too). Among these grasping neurons for precision grip, there were some that activated when the monkey did not move at all, but simply watched somebody else grasping a tiny object (not necessarily a raisin, but any kind of tiny object) with a precision grip. The activity of these cells nearly suggested that while watching other people busy with their own activities, the monkey appeared to be seeing her own actions reflected by a mirror. Hence, the scientists decided to call these brain cells mirror neurons (Gallese et al., 1996).

The early studies on mirror neurons focused on the brain region in which these cells were originally discovered. These early studies demonstrated that there are two main classes of mirror neurons. While approximately one-third of mirror neurons activated for exactly the same action, whether performed or observed (these are called strictly congruent mirror neurons), about two-thirds of mirror neurons also fired for other kinds of observed actions (these are called broadly congruent mirror neurons) (Gallese et al., 1996). These neurons would activate as long as the observed action achieved the same goal of the performed action. This property suggests that these cells implement a fairly sophisticated mapping of the perceived actions of other people onto the motor repertoire of the perceiver. But how sophisticated is this mapping? Studies have shown that mirror neurons can activate for observed actions that are not completely in sight (that is, vision is partially occluded) (Umilta et al., 2001) and for simply listening to the sound of the action (e.g., breaking a peanut) (Kohler et al., 2002). The most compelling of these studies demonstrate that the majority of mirror neurons do not even code the action itself (e.g., grasping), but rather the intention associated with it (e.g., grasping to eat rather than grasping to place in a container) (Fogassi et al., 2005).

All these data suggest that when we watch other people's activities, mirror neurons automatically make our own motor system active as if we are performing those activities. This seems a wonderfully efficient mechanism for imitation, which is a fundamental behavior for learning and transmission of culture, and possibly for empathy. However, the mirror mechanism in the brain also suggests that we are automatically influenced by what we perceive, thus proposing a plausible neurobiological mechanism for contagion of violent behavior.

Recent Developments in Mirror Neuron Research

While the early studies on mirror neurons focused on hand and mouth actions, more recent studies have demonstrated the existence of mirror neurons for other kinds of actions (or specific aspects of the observed action) and most importantly in many brain regions. This new wave of studies suggests that the neural mirror mechanism is rather diffuse and pervasive.

In monkeys, three different labs have reported mirror neurons for reaching movements in two different brain areas (Cisek and Kalaska, 2004; Pfeifer et al., 2008; Dushanova and Donoghue, 2010). Mirror neurons have also been reported for eye movements (Shepherd et al., 2009). The neurons that code for eye movements tend to have a preferred direction. That is, some neurons activate for eye movements toward a specific sector of space, but not others. Mirror neurons for eye movements do the same. When the monkey is simply watching another monkey looking in the preferred direction of the neuron, the neuron activates as if the monkey was moving the eyes toward that direction. This mirroring mechanism may be important for gaze following and joint attention, two foundational behaviors for the development of social cognition.

Single-cell recordings require invasive brain surgical procedures and are obviously performed in experimental animals, but not in human subjects volunteering for research experiments. However, in some rather exceptional situations, it is possible to piggy-back on existing medical procedures to obtain recordings of individual cells in the human brain. A recent study indeed was able to do so (Mukamel et al., 2010). The subjects of the study were patients with epilepsy who did not respond well to medications. In these situations, it is appropriate to treat epilepsy with brain surgery, in which the neurosurgeon removes the pathological brain tissue and spares the healthy tissue. To determine the epileptic focus or foci, the surgeon implants depth electrodes into the brain. While in the hospital, the patient stops taking medications and eventually seizes, thus allowing the electrodes implanted in the depth of the brain to show the surgeon exactly where the pathological brain tissue is.

Typically, this procedure only requires the registration of the electroencephalograph (EEG) signal that allows the surgeon to localize the affected tissue. However, with a slight modification of the electrodes used for this procedure, it is also possible to record the activity of individual neurons from the brain of patients. A recent study that recorded for the first time individual mirror neurons in humans reported mirror neurons in two areas that were previously not known to have these kinds of brain cells (Mukamel

et al., 2010). Note that the location of the electrodes in the study on neurosurgical patients is exclusively dictated by medical considerations, not
by research questions. Thus, the study in human neurosurgical patients did
not record at all from brain areas in which mirror neurons were found in
the monkey brain. The two areas in which mirror neurons in humans were
found are known to be important for initiating action and for memory. Mirror neurons in a brain region known to be important for memory suggest
that we mirror the actions of others in a rather rich fashion. That is, when
I watch somebody else grasping a cup of coffee, my brain not only mirrors
the motor plans to perform the same action, but also retrieves memory
traces of my previous grasping actions. This neural mechanism provides
an "inner imitation" of the behavior of other people, which most likely
allows us to learn by observation and imitation, and to empathize with
others. However, it also makes us more prone to imitate what we see, thus
facilitating social contagion.

The Study of the Mirror Neuron
System with Noninvasive Techniques

So far we have discussed data from single-cell recordings in monkeys
and, in one study, in humans. These data are probably the most compelling data one can obtain in neuroscience. However, single-cell recordings
require invasive brain surgery, and their use in humans is obviously extremely limited. There is a large body of scientific literature on the study
of mirror neurons in humans that uses noninvasive forms of brain investigation. The four main techniques used are functional magnetic resonance
imaging (Iacoboni et al., 2005), EEG (Oberman et al., 2007), magneto-
encephalography (Hari et al., 1998), and transcranial magnetic stimulation
(Fadiga et al., 1995; Aziz-Zadeh et al., 2002). Although the data obtained
with these techniques are not as compelling as the data obtained with
single-cell recordings, they are still extremely valuable. These techniques
make it possible to study healthy subjects and neuropsychiatric patients,
and to correlate the activity recorded in the brain with behavioral variables.

The data from this vast literature seem to confirm the initial intuitions
about the role of mirror neurons in social behavior. Human brain areas
with mirroring properties have been associated with imitation (Iacoboni et
al., 1999) and empathy (Carr et al., 2003). Indeed, some studies show cor-
relations between individual differences in empathy and activity in mirror
neuron areas (Pfeifer et al., 2008). The more empathic the subject is, the
higher the activity during imitation (Pfeifer et al., 2008), or simply during
observation of actions (Kaplan and Iacoboni, 2006) or emotional facial
expressions of other people (Pfeifer et al., 2008), including pain (Avenanti et
al., 2005). Furthermore, patients who find social interactions difficult, such

as patients with autism spectrum disorders, seem to show reduced activity in mirror neuron areas (Dapretto et al., 2006). These data support the idea that mirror neurons are important for the effortless, automatic understanding of the mental states of other people (Iacoboni, 2009), and may also be the basis of automatic imitation (Cross and Iacoboni, 2011).

Control of Mirroring to Prevent Contagion of Violence

If we have a mechanism in the brain that automatically activates our own motor system when we see others performing actions, we should also have a control mechanism to avoid continuous automatic imitation. Indeed, while humans tend to imitate others automatically and subconsciously, they tend to do that in a subtle way, imitating postures or the onset of movements (when I reach for the glass you may reach for the napkin), without overtly parroting the behavior of other people. Our behavior would be highly dysfunctional if we were imitating each other all the time. For instance, even during conversation humans tend to imitate each other, often using the same grammatical structures or noun selection (if we are talking about furniture in the living room and I say sofa, it is highly unlikely that the person talking to me will use a synonym like couch; that person most likely will also use the word sofa) (Garrod and Pickering, 2004; Pickering and Garrod, 2007). However, we do not repeat word for word what the other person has just told us. What are the mechanisms and neural systems for control of mirroring?

The evidence, albeit not conclusive yet, points to a number of potential mechanisms for control of mirroring. Neurological patients with prefrontal lesions show imitative behavior, the rather dysfunctional tendency to imitate whatever other people do in front of them. The lesions that produce this rare behavior are very large, suggesting that multiple brain centers may be involved in mirroring control (Lhermitte et al., 1986; De Renzi et al., 1996). Some imaging studies indeed suggest that multiple brain areas in the frontal lobe may implement some type of control of mirroring (Brass et al., 2005; Bien et al., 2009). The differential role of these areas is unclear. Finally, other imaging data suggest that in some situations control is implemented by reconfiguring the connectivity among many different brain systems important for sensory-motor behavior (Cross and Iacoboni, 2011).

The study of the mechanisms of control of mirroring is potentially extremely important. If we can understand how the brain implements control of mirroring, we can in principle intervene and modulate its activity. In some cases, as in the case of autism, it may be beneficial to reduce control and increase mirroring. In some other cases, as in the case of individuals exposed to violent behavior who may be involved in spreading contagion of violence, it may be beneficial to increase control of mirroring, thus reducing imitative violence and possibly preventing the spreading of contagion of violence (Iacoboni, 2008).

Conclusions

Mirror neurons provide an important missing link between the social science data on contagion of violence and the model that draws similarities between contagious mechanisms in infectious diseases and contagion of violence. They provide a neurobiologically grounded mechanism that is fairly automatic and reflexive (albeit not entirely reflexive, of course). It is important to pay attention to the neuroscience data because they suggest forms of human automatic behavior that require careful consideration when planning interventions and policy that attempt to reduce contagion of violence.

II.6

CONTAGION OF VIOLENCE

Eleanor Taylor-Nicholson, L.L.M.
and
Barry Krisberg, Ph.D.
Earl Warren Institute on Law and Social Policy at the
University of California, Berkeley, School of Law

Among justice system officials and the citizenry at large, one of the most accepted methods for dealing with individual and community violence is punishment of offenders through incarceration. The United States has the largest imprisonment rate of any nation. As of the end of 2011, 2.3 million people (one in 33 adults) were in correctional facilities, either at the state, federal, or county level. The majority of violent offenders are sentenced to prison (BJS, 2011). Besides these adults, more than 75,000 juveniles were held in juvenile incarceration facilities or adult institutions.

The role of prisons in responding to violent crime has grown considerably. In 2008, the number of offenders sentenced to state prison for violent offenses reached 715,400, up from 95,400 violent offenders in 2000. This increase accounted for 60 percent of prison growth during this period (BJS, 2011).

Little is understood, however, about whether prisons really work to reduce or prevent the spread of violence in society. Many people assume that prison prevents violence, at least temporarily, by keeping violent individuals off the street. But what if imprisonment makes matters worse and increases transmission? Few longitudinal studies have examined the effects of incarceration as a factor in the mental and physical health of former prisoners, let alone more nuanced analyses such as the effects of particular types of incarceration facilities or length of imprisonment.

We do know that recidivism is high among former inmates, and we also have some limited indication from studies of prison life about the levels and types of violence among prisoners and former inmates. It is striking that this literature may suggest that incarceration could in fact exacerbate violence in some cases, both within the prison walls and in the broader community. This raises significant questions about the dominant ideology that determines how governments invest in strategies to reduce violence.

Violence in Prisons

"[P]rison is no fairy-tale world. He never said who did it, but we all knew. Things went on like that for awhile. . . . Every so often; Andy would show up with fresh bruises. The Sisters kept at him—sometimes he was able to fight 'em off, sometimes not." —The Shawshank Redemption

One big concern about addressing violence through incarceration is that prisons themselves are extremely violent places. While this has long been recognized, quantitative studies only began in the 1970s (Ellis et al., 1974) and epidemiological research more recently has allowed us to better understand the frequency and characteristics of violence in facilities.

Nancy Wolff and Jing Shi, for example, have conducted research in prisons across a northeastern state of the United States to determine frequency of victimization of physical and sexual violence. They defined physical violence in line with the National Violence Against Women and Men surveys to include being hit, slapped, kicked, bit, choked, beat up, or hit with or threatened with a weapon. Of the 20,447 inmates at 14 facilities (13 for males and one for females) surveyed, Wolff and Shi (2009) found that approximately 20 percent of female inmates and 25 percent of male inmates reported being physically assaulted during their current sentence by either another inmate or a guard. In the previous 6 months before the survey, men reported much higher incidence of assault with a weapon than women, and also reported much higher victimization by a staff member; nearly one in four men was assaulted by a staff member in the 6-month period.

Not all prisoners are violent, and not all inmates are victimized. On average, victims in the Wolff and Shi study were in their early 30s, African American, had spent at least 2 years in the facility, had 4 to 5 years remaining to serve, and had spent 8 years in prison since turning 18 (Wolff and Shi, 2009). Victimization was noted to depend on age and vulnerability. Younger inmates were more likely to be targeted either by other inmates (one in three younger inmates was assaulted by another inmate during their sentence compared to one in four among older inmates) or by a corrections officer (36 versus 25 percent). Furthermore, sexual orientation and mental illness/disability were identified as contributing to prison sexual assault in one quarter of all assaults by other inmates.

Other research has demonstrated the powerful "situational" impact of prisons on prisoner and guard behavior. Of these, the most famous is the Stanford Prison Simulation study by Philip Zimbardo and colleagues. In 1971, Professor Zimbardo engaged a group of "normal, average, healthy American college males" in a planned 2-week simulation of a prison. The researchers assigned half of the students to role-play "guards" and rotated on 8-hour shifts, and the other half to play "prisoners" continuously. After just 1 week the project had to be terminated because "it became apparent that many of the 'prisoners' were in serious distress and many of the guards were behaving in ways that brutalized and degraded their fellow subjects." The prisoners demonstrated "learned helplessness" behavior and the guards displayed physical and verbal aggressiveness that was not indicated in their preexperiment personality tests.

Juvenile facilities are not immune from these challenges. Mendel (2011) conducted an analysis of the court-sanctioned remedies ordered to address violent or abusive conditions in juvenile facilities, as well as of reports written by reputable media outlets. The Annie E. Casey Foundation found there had been documented "systemic violence, abuse and/or excessive use of isolation or restraints," as opposed to isolated incidents, in a number of states, plus the District of Columbia and Puerto Rico. The findings are as follows: since 1970, 39 states; since 1990, 32 states, and since 2000, 22 states.

Root Causes Left Untreated

The causes of violent behavior are rarely treated effectively in prisons. A number of researchers have argued, for example, that prison violence may often be related to untreated mental illness. Emotionally disturbed inmates or inmates who require mental health services have been found to commit prison infractions disproportionately compared to other inmates. Because the correlation between prison infractions and violence is often high, these inmates are disproportionately involved in violent incidents as well (James and Glaze, 2006).

Preexisting mental illness is not limited to adult inmates. In one early study of juveniles, 85 boys detained in California for mostly violent offenses were given a standard psychiatric screen, a semi-structured interview for posttraumatic stress disorder (PTSD), and self-report questionnaires measuring personality traits and defenses. A sex- and age-matched group was used for comparing psychometrics. The results indicated that 32 percent of the inmates fulfilled criteria for PTSD, and 20 percent partial criteria. Half of the subjects said witnessing of interpersonal violence was the traumatizing event (Steiner et al., 1997), indicating the vulnerability of these incarcerated youth to exposure to violence.

Incarceration may in some cases exacerbate mental illness or emotional frailty of inmates. Craig Haney, also one of the researchers in the Zimbardo experiment, has subsequently written further about the psychological impact of incarceration (Haney, 2002), and identified the following common symptoms among his clients:

- dependence on institution, loss of capacity/judgment;
- hypervigilance, distrust, suspicion;
- emotional over-control, alienation, and psychological distancing;
- social withdrawal and isolation;
- incorporation of exploitative norms; and
- diminished sense of self-worth and personal value.

Importantly, Haney notes that these effects vary from individual to individual, and may not necessarily be permanent. This echoes another considerable body of research that has explored the ways different prisoners adjust to life in prison and noted that some prisoners even improve functioning (Bukstel and Kilman, 1980). A Canadian study found that some prisoners saw being in prison as a chance to turn their lives around, and many inmates, while resenting imprisonment, expected their lives to improve after release (Zamble and Porprino, 1988). There is little research on the attributes of prisons that are helpful or hurtful in terms of postrelease adjustment. An assumption has been that smaller prisons, which have more education and treatment services and less restrictive custody situations, are less criminogenic, but the research on these issues still needs to be conducted.

Release and Reentry

Of all those incarcerated in U.S. prisons, more than 93 percent will return home eventually; more than 700,000 persons are released from prisons each year (see, generally, Travis and Waul, 2003). However, recidivism rates are high. One study found that within 3 years, 67 percent of returning prisoners were rearrested for a serious offense and 52 percent were returned to prison for a new criminal offense (Langan and Levin, 2002). These rates are highest for nonviolent criminals (robbery, burglary, larceny, motor vehicle theft), but violent criminals also recidivate. Overall, 1990s data showed that released prisoners had at least a 53 times higher homicide rate than the general population (Langan and Levin, 2002).[5]

Some evidence has also emerged of high levels of family violence among current and recently released inmates. White et al. (2002) reported that 1 in 3 men incarcerated in federal prisons for *low-risk crimes* admitted recent physical violence against intimate female partners and 1 in 10 reported severe violence toward women. Other studies have found that domestic violence perpetrated by recently released inmates was related to frustration at joblessness, changed relationship circumstances, and displaced anger at incarceration (Oliver and Hairston, 2008).

Conclusion

Although there is good reason to assume that sources of violence transmission spread violence among prisoners, family members, the children of prisons, and in the communities where released inmates return, the research on this key topic is underdeveloped. What longitudinal studies are available rarely employ the experience of incarceration as an independent variable. The criminal justice community assumes that incapacitation is the major tool to stop violence in society. Incarceration consumes an enormous amount of government funds in lieu of spending on community-based violence prevention programming.

With the movement away from a pure criminal justice model to one that is informed by public health principles, the primacy of imprisonment will need to be reevaluated. In the past, other public health issues, such as tuberculosis, polio, mental illness, and HIV, were responded to with incapacitation and isolation of affected individuals. This approach was not very effective in terms of curtailing the problems in the community.

We need much rigorous research on the ways in which the prison experience increases exposure to violence both within and outside the walls. There is an urgent need to examine how prisons and reentry programs can be redesigned to stem the contagion of violence.

---

[5] Of the 272,111 prisoners released in 1994, 719 were rearrested for homicide in 13 states in 1995, 8.4 percent of all the homicides in those states.

II.7

NATIVE ASPIRATIONS: ADDRESSING THE CONTAGION OF VIOLENCE IN THE CONTEXT OF HISTORICAL TRAUMA

Iris PrettyPaint, Ph.D.
and
Corinne Taylor
Native Aspirations

Background

For the past 7 years, an innovative and transformative project called Native Aspirations (NA) has successfully addressed the crisis of youth violence in American Indian and Alaskan Native (AI/AN) communities. Sixty-five Native communities across some of the most remote and underserved areas of the United States have benefited from the NA approach. Native Aspirations started in 2005 with emergency funding from the Substance Abuse and Mental Health Services Administration (SAMHSA), the aim of which was to tackle the violence facing AI/AN youth. The NA approach respects tribal sovereignty by collaborating with tribal leaders, community members, and tribal behavioral health departments. At the heart of the NA approach is the recognition of two salient factors that contribute to both the problem of and the solutions to community-wide violence. The first factor is the role that historical trauma plays in community violence. The second factor consists of honoring the local knowledge and cultural practices that heal communities.

The traumatic history of war, colonization, removal, and oppression of indigenous populations in the United States is well documented. As a result of this trauma, the American Indian population, which was 15-60 million before European contact, dropped to its lowest level, just under 200,000, at the turn of the 20th century (Thornton, 1987; Campbell, 2010). While the population has grown, with just over 7 million people identifying as AI/AN (alone and mixed race) in the 2010 Census, the effects of trauma can still be seen in the violence, poverty, and behavioral health indicators in Native populations.

Effects of Historical Trauma

The effects of trauma on the lives of AI/ANs have been examined and discussed in the historical trauma literature. Historical trauma can include the loss of language, spiritual practices, ceremonies, and lifestyle caused by forcible removal from traditional homelands, federal relocation policies, and paternalistic practices. AI/AN children were forcibly separated from their families and communities and placed in boarding schools, ostensibly to educate them, but the true objective was to "erase and replace" Indian culture (Trafzer et al., 2006).

Historical trauma is defined as the cumulative emotional and psychological wounding over the lifespan and across generations, caused by massive group trauma. It can be characterized by violence that is both individually and systemically perpetrated on individuals, families, and systems that are without mechanisms in place to cope with repeated traumatic events (Yellow Horse Brave Heart, 2003). By this definition, AI/AN communities continue to experience historical trauma today. A small but growing body of research is beginning to conceptualize and measure the effects of historical trauma on AI/AN communities (Whitbeck et al., 2004).

Institutional Cofactors

Although the heartbreaking statistics for AI/AN psychosocial cofactors of violence are easy to obtain, they must be considered in the context of the systemic and institutional cofactors, which are more difficult to quantify. Across Indian country, the roles of courts, police, and incarceration facilities are multicultural, multi-institutional, and multijurisdictional (Champagne, 2012). Jurisdictional and systemic complexities can lead to frustration, desensitization, and hopelessness when it comes to addressing change in AI/AN communities. The complexities of these institutional cofactors make causation difficult to attribute. This confusion of causation can lead to split perspectives in addressing the problems of violence. Some people believe the tribal court personnel need more training; others see the vast distances police are asked to patrol as the cause; still others see the enabling roles families play as contributors to the violence. These multiple perspectives are difficult to bridge in terms of prevention. A tribal prosecutor from one of our communities said, "People are desensitized to the issues of rape, incest, and domestic violence and don't see how their actions hurt others."

The NA approach works within the tribal infrastructure to strengthen interagency coordination and collaboration. For example, two NA communities that have historically not worked together, but whose youth attend the same high school, have recently begun collaborating on prevention activities. Another NA strategy is to encourage communities to mentor each other. Communities have responded positively to this strategy by planning and conducting prevention activities together.

Psychosocial Cofactors

The far-reaching web created by historical and current trauma that traps AI/AN communities includes the ongoing legacy of both institutional and psychosocial cofactors. Across Indian country, the high incidence of violence, suicide, substance abuse, and mental health disorders is well documented. Each of these behavioral health issues, which are at rates twice that of the general population, feed into the contagion of violence for tribal communities. On average, American Indians experience 1 violent crime for every 10 residents age 12 or older. Although violent crime rates were significantly higher in every age group under 35, for ages 25 to 34 they are 2.5 times higher than the U.S. general population (DOJ, 2011). According to the National Crime Victimization Survey, AI/AN rates of violent victimization are two times that of the next highest group (black non-Hispanic) and nearly four times higher than the average of the other three groups (white non-Hispanic, Hispanic, and Asian and Pacific Islander) (DOJ, 2011). This violence and victimization have a devastating impact on youth, families, schools, and communities.

These numbers do not fully capture the tremendous psychological and physical toll that sexual assault, domestic violence, rape, and posttraumatic stress disorder (PTSD) take on youth and families (HHS, 2011). Amnesty International's interviews with survivors, activists, and support workers across the United States suggest that available statistics greatly underestimate the severity of the problem. For example, on one reservation, many of the women who agreed to be interviewed could not think of any Native women within their community who had not been subjected to sexual violence (Amnesty International, 1997). In addition, in one population of American Indian adolescents, 61 percent of children had witnessed at least one traumatic event (Jones et al., 1997). PTSD is an anxiety disorder characterized by a fight-or-flight response that becomes triggered when, after having experienced a life-threatening event, a person responds repeatedly with the same reactions to minor stimuli, even when their life is not in danger. Because violence in some form is the typical trigger for this condition, the PTSD rates can be seen as a gauge for the contagion of violence. Obviously, when one is continually responding as if in a life-threatening situation, problem solving, decision making, and a sense of belonging are impacted.

With these staggering rates of community violence, comorbid youth suicide and bullying have emerged as significant issues and priorities for AI/AN communities. Suicide is the second leading cause of death among Indian youth between ages 15 and 24—1.8 times higher than the national average. When clusters occur, the suicide rate in a community can soar to 10 times the national average. Among AI/AN youth, suicide is the second leading cause of death behind accidental injuries (HHS, 2010). Tragically, Alaska Natives commit suicide at rates four times the national average. For Alaska Native males of all ages, the suicide rate is six times higher than the national average, with teen suicide rates nearly six times the rate of non-AI/AN teens (Statewide Suicide Prevention Council, 2004). A National

Education Association study released in 2011, *Focus on American Indians and Alaskan Natives: The Scourge of Suicides Among American Indian and Alaska Native Youth*, strongly suggests that bullying is one of the contributing factors in the high rate of suicides among American Indians and Alaska Natives.

The most recent Indian Health Service *Trends* publication states that the AI/AN alcohol-related death rate is 519 percent greater than the U.S. all-races rate (HHS, 2011). Risk of exposure to violence and risk of experiencing multiple victimization episodes is higher when family alcohol problems or drug use are present (Stevens et al., 2005; Hanson et al., 2006). Chief of the Blackfeet Nation Earl Old Person states, "These statistics haunt our communities and touch each of our lives. The pain our communities endure as a result of generations of active and passive assault upon our land, language, spiritual practices, ceremonies, and traditional lifestyle is real. Today that nightmare has a name: historical trauma."

Native Aspirations Approach

In 2005, SAMHSA contracted with Kauffman and Associates, Inc., to create a nationwide tribal community movement toward healing, violence prevention, and positive youth development. Employing a team of AI/AN mental health professionals, the NA project staff first consults with the local tribal government of the targeted community to confirm their willingness to participate. A central focus of the NA approach is recognizing the sovereignty of each community and supporting their choices about how to connect to young people. In turn, the project provides opportunities for youth to share, discuss, and understand the difficult challenges they confront. NA understands the importance of creating and fostering safe environments for young people to process and understand trauma while creating a vision for a better, healthier community. These environments are created by modeling traditional values, such as respect and sharing, while also embracing digital technology to create visual stories that preserve and convey their vision of hope and strength for the future.

NA begins work in each community by organizing a large community healing ceremony known as the GONA (Gathering of Native Americans) or GOAN (Gathering of Alaska Natives) to support open dialogue about historical trauma, conduct an inventory of community needs, and enhance connections among organizations and individuals already working on violence prevention. This team approach has a demonstrable impact on creating a community-wide prevention strategy that involves everyone. "Native Aspirations provides us with continual support, bringing valuable new tools to the table and helping us to learn what other tribes are doing successfully," said Myrna Warrington, council member of Menominee Nation.

NA encourages AI/AN communities to bring culture-based prevention strategies to the development of community-based prevention planning. The NA approach focuses on empowering planning and interventions in the following ways: (1) encourage the expression of cultural norms and values, (2) bridge evidence-based interventions (EBIs) and cultural practices, and (3) enhance capacity of local community members in key sustainability skills.

Cultural norms, values, and beliefs provide the informal social controls that counteract antisocial behavior, which relates to levels of community violence (Sampson et al., 2002). Levels of community violence not only contribute to youth violence and bullying, but also are a risk factor in mental, emotional, and behavioral disorders (IOM, 2009). Therefore, impacting these informal social controls should affect rates of suicide and suicidal behavior. Through events based on local culture and existing resources (e.g., the community mapping and readiness assessment event, the GONA/GOAN, the community prevention planning event), communities review their strengths; articulate cultural values in a public forum that connects elders, adults, and youth; and collaboratively create a plan for prevention activities and sustainability. Native Aspirations encourages communities, as a part of their prevention plans, to integrate community-sponsored cultural intervention activities, such as drum groups, culture camps, cultural skills building, and autobiographical digital films about cultural values.

Nearly all EBIs for violence, bullying, and suicide prevention were evaluated using non-Native populations. Often EBIs do not take into account cultural norms outside the dominant culture or disallow adaptation to various linguistic and cultural frameworks or value systems. For example, the suicide intervention Question Persuade Refer (QPR) encourages and trains laypersons to recognize and respond to suicide warning signs by asking about suicide. However, the QPR approach does not consider AI/AN cultural taboos against explicitly talking about suicide, which hold that speaking about suicide attracts it to you. In response to the need for culturally competent suicide prevention programming, NA has developed and disseminated materials regarding culturally adapting EBIs to tribal communities. For communities that have created their own culturally based interventions, NA assists them in validating and replicating cultural practices so they can meet the standards set for establishing a cultural intervention as a promising or best practice, potentially for use or adaptation across other AI/AN communities.

Lastly, NA's training and technical assistance focuses on building capacity in skills that are fundamental for sustainability: planning, collaboration, self-determination, and evaluation. Oppression and cultural suppression have undermined these skills, which once had to exist for AI/AN cultures to survive. The unique difference in the NA approach is that each community is treated with respect, consulted in advance, and empowered to seek its solutions. Instead of imposing practices based on predetermined criteria or competition, the project training and technical assistance support focus on building on existing community strengths, local agencies, and personnel.

The underlying philosophy of NA is that the answers to the challenges facing Native youth are found within the cultural traditions, teachings, and stories of their families and communities. Based on our experience and anecdotal evidence, we believe the NA approach strengthens cultural protective factors, helps to heal historical trauma, and thus breaks the cycle of violence. Those of us who care about the survival of AI/AN tribes—and the future generations—need to come together to heal the wounds of historical trauma.

II.8

CONTAGION OF VIOLENCE AGAINST REFUGEE WOMEN IN MIGRATION AND DISPLACEMENT

Fariyal Ross-Sheriff, Ph.D.
Howard University School of Social Work

Women are vulnerable to violence during times of migration and displacement, specifically where social structures are disintegrated by war. Two groups that are most vulnerable to violence are female refugees and internally displaced women (IDW) among displaced populations. A refugee woman is someone who flees her country to escape war or persecution based on race, religion, gender, ethnicity, and political orientation (UNHCR, 1992). IDW are those who are still in their country, but have fled from their home place for the same reasons—war or persecution. Of the total refugee populations, more than 80 percent are women and their dependent children. The numbers of IDW are higher than refugees and they experience high levels of violence. Because the incidents are underreported, the true scale of the problem is generally unknown. Gender-based violence against refugee women and IDW is a serious human rights abuse and a public health issue because of its substantial consequences for women's physical, mental, and reproductive health problems.

Gender-based violence has been defined as narrowly as rape, or broadly to include physical, mental, and emotional abuse. The General Assembly of the United Declaration of Violence Against Women defined it broadly, as any act of violence that results or is likely to result in physical, sexual, or mental harm or suffering to women, including threats of coercion or arbitrary deprivation of liberty whether occurring in public or private life

(United Nations, 1993). Refugee women and IDW incur gender-based violence in many forms and from diverse sources ranging from family members and people who are supposed to protect them, such as police and refugee administrators, to total strangers. Amnesty International (1997, 2008) has reported especially dire conditions for IDW in several African conflict areas, including Republic of Congo, Sudan, and Uganda. In their 2008 *Special Report on Sexual Violence in the Democratic Republic of Congo (DRC)*, Tosh and Chazan report epidemic repeated violence against girls and women in the eastern part of the DRC. Similarly, *Lives Blown Apart: Crimes Against Women in Times of Conflict* reports thousands of Congolese women and girls suffering repeated bodily harm and by different forces (Amnesty International, 2004). Among the crimes against women and girls are repeated experiences, during and after the rapes, of tortures and bodily harm, including vagina mutilation with spears, machetes, sticks, broken bottles, and gun barrels; and cutting off breasts, clitoris, and vaginal lips with razor blades. The pain and suffering from such heinous crimes take years to heal for those who survive, and leave many with physical handicaps and emotional turmoil for the rest of their lives.

This paper examines the violence that refugees and IDW experience in terms of the transmission of violence during the five stages of migration and displacement. It also considers how violence can be stopped and women supported to overcome the trauma of violence in safe spaces with support from service providers, family, and friends. The five stages of displacement and migration from pre-uprooting to adaptation, as described by a model developed by Cox (1987) and Berry (2001), are

1. pre-uprooting/preflight in countries of origin;
2. uprooting when they flee their homes to avoid persecution;
3. transition in refugee camps, camps for internally displaced persons (IDPs), or as self-settled refugees in countries of first asylum;
4. resettlement in countries of first asylum or to a second country of asylum or repatriation after the end of war; and
5. adaptation and integration to a new homeland.

Uprooting and displacement involves multiple losses and experiences of violence, issues of trauma, and consequent physical and mental health problems for refugee women and IDW. Refugee women and IDW can be supported to overcome or at least mitigate negative health effects if they receive appropriate support from health and mental health specialists, family, friends, and community during the stages of resettlement and adaptation (Ross-Sheriff et al., 2012).

Preuprooting

During the preuprooting stage in times of war, women are vulnerable to increasing domestic violence from spouses and relatives due to stress, availability of arms, and depletion of resources. Women's risks are increased when the households' men flee or leave to join fighting forces and women stay back to protect their children and manage their homes (Jansen et al., 2004). They incur violence by fighters from both sides, as described by Waldman (2005), who reports widespread atrocities where women's bodies become battlegrounds. Rapes, kidnapping, and sexual servitude are common in war (Rehn and Sirleaf, 2002; Wood, 2004). Some are victims of gang rapes and suffer from physical injuries; sexually transmitted diseases, including HIV/AIDS; and miscarriages. Women have to remain silent after being raped or violated lest their spouses reject them and other family members abuse them for bringing shame to the family and their community ostracizes them. This worsens the mental and physical harm. Conflicts in such places as Bosnia, Liberia, Rwanda, and Sierra Leone have drawn attention to the modern use of rape as a weapon of war.

Uprooting/Flight

The uprooting stage involves flight from the refugees' and IDW's homes to a location far away in their own country or to another country. Women experience several forms of severe anxiety and violence during flight, including constant fear of being discovered and robbed of their few possessions; pain of seeing children and spouses being physically assaulted; and personal injury, molestation, and gang rapes inflicted by police, armed forces, and armed bandits. Despite the atrocities and suffering, women have to continue to provide daily care for their children and families. As is the case during preuprooting, the violation of women's bodily and sexual integrity is compounded by the victims' reluctance to report rape for fear of family shame and community ostracism. They consider discussion regarding molestation and rape as shameful and so they suffer in silence. Many believe it would have been better if they were killed rather than raped. For them the disgrace from rape is a violation of their integrity, both in religious and social terms.

Transition

During this third stage of forced migration, refugee women and IDW either live in refugee or IDP camps or self-settle, doubling up with families and friends in countries of first asylum, or at a safer location in their own country. Women may experience temporary feelings of relief from having successfully managed to leave life-threatening and very challenging conditions. However, these feelings of relief soon pass and are replaced by feelings of uncertainty, fear, and anxiety.

Women and children make up 80 percent of the refugees worldwide. Refugee camps have overcrowded conditions, unsanitary facilities, inadequate health care, and lack of food, compounded by lack of safety and security from physical, emotional, and mental abuse, especially for women and children (Cole et al., 1993). Among the most pressing challenges in the camps reported by Chung were a "lack of physical safety, lawlessness, violence, the lack of effective law enforcement and internal security" (Chung, 2001, p. 117). Mollica (1986) noted that 95 percent of the Cambodian women in refugee camps had experiences of unwanted sexual encounters, abuse, or rape.

Refugee women and IDW are responsible for day-to-day survival of their families in the camps and self-settle temporary locations. They must collect, find, and carry fuel for cooking and water; prepare food; and attend to the health, safety, and other basic needs of the family. Physicians for Human Rights, in partnership with Harvard initiative, noted that Darfuri women did not feel safe in Chad. They were in constant fear of being raped and subsequently rejected by their husbands and ostracized by their families; yet, they had to leave camps to gather wood for fuel to cook food. They had to endure an oppressive environment of insecurity on a daily basis. Camps commonly have lit sanitary latrines, but women often do not use them at night as they are vulnerable to attack by refugee men as they walk from their shelter to the latrine location. Amnesty International (2004) reported that women of refugee camps are raped each day while collecting water. Some refugee women are forced to exchange sex for protection by the police officers and other male camp residents. The mental impacts of such oppressive conditions include high levels of anxiety and depression among women.

Resettlement

The resettlement stage begins when the refugees or IDW are cleared for repatriation back to their homeland or accepted for permanent settlement in the first country of asylum or in a second or third country of asylum. The plans for permanent resettlement or repatriation are generally developed by the Office of the United Nations High Commissioner for Refugees or by a nongovernmental organization. Women refugees and IDW and their families generally receive at least some support for resettlement or repatriation and for rebuilding their lives. This may include assistance to build new homes or to rebuild their former homes, which are often destroyed. The support can include help with housing, food, water, education, health care, and income generation. However, women continue to experience severe challenges from lack of employment, poverty, and racial discrimination after resettlement (Gozdiak and Long, 2005). They survive and rebuild their lives (Gozdiak and Long, 2005). The potential for violence continues at home in the form of domestic violence and aggression in the community for many women.

In the United States, like several western resettlement countries, agencies such as the U.S. Committee for Immigrants and Refugees, Church World Service, Episcopal Migration Ministries, International Rescue Committee, Lutheran Immigration and Refugee Service, U.S. Catholic Conference, and World Relief Corporation, provide services for predeparture assistance, medical examinations, U.S. culture orientation, assistance with housing, school enrollment of children, English language training, and health insurance. The services are designed to facilitate resettlement, with a focus on acculturation and adaptation to the new homeland. However, mental health conditions arising from past trauma may impede the progress of refugee women to adjust to a new country; to develop a supportive community; and to navigate the economic, educational, political, and social services.

Adaptation and Integration

This last stage of migration involves settling back home for repatriated women or in the host country for resettled women, adapting and integrating into the structures of the society, and eventually learning to lead normal lives. Refugee women and their families experience discrimination, and cultural and language differences as they start their lives in a host country. Such experiences can impede their ability to establish new friendship networks and support systems, leading to long-standing feelings of alienation and loneliness (Potocky-Tripodi, 2002). Discrimination is recognized as an adverse mental health risk for the refugees in general and for refugee women, in particular (Finch et al., 2000). Discrimination and microaggression in adaptation stage may not only originate from the people of the host countries, but also from other refugees from their own countries who had arrived earlier (Sue, 2010). Additionally, cultural differences create stress for refugee women, especially where the culture of origin is distinctly different from the culture of the country of resettlement. Martin (2004) notes that refugee women heads of household, single women, or widowed women are especially at risk of health and mental health problems, which are exacerbated by language barriers in the new country. However, over time most do learn the host language and manage well. In a survey of refugees living in the United States who came from Africa, Eastern Europe, and Russia, 90 percent spoke no or little English at the time of arrival, but within 5 years 68 percent spoke English well or fluently (Martin, 2004). It is generally believed that refugee women learn English language at a slower pace than men because they are socially more isolated in host society than men.

Gozdziak (2009) discusses a number of challenges faced by resettled refugee women, including the difficulty of making "life-and-death decisions at every stage of the migration process" (Gozdziak, 2009, p. 146) and the mental health consequences that must be acknowledged during resettlement. She notes that resettled refugee women are resilient and she recommends an inclusive model of addressing health and mental health needs, using cultural-specific methods of coping and surviving traumatic experiences such as indigenous healing, religion, and spirituality.

In her analysis of the day-to-day living situations and experiences of institutionalized practices with Afghan refugee women resettled in Canada and repatriated in Afghanistan, Dossa notes serious mental health problems, including anxiety, alienation, and severe depression. However, these women want to build a new life in their host or home countries (Dossa, 2004, 2010). They want to work. They want to leave their past sufferings and dehumanizing experiences behind; and, most importantly, they want to work toward a future for themselves and their children. However, lack of opportunities, gendered discrimination, marginalization, and insensitive bureaucratic and institutional responses intensify their pain rather than provide support to overcome the impact of past trauma. Dossa suggests a holistic approach to develop survival and coping strategies involving family, community, and social support for women and their children.

Violence against refugee women and IDW is a serious problem that can be deterred, mitigated, and redressed through prevention and intervention programs in all locations, including countries of origin, refugee and IDP camps, and countries of resettlement. Prevention will require conditions of safety and security in countries of origin, and development and implementation of laws within a civil society. Interventions will require educational and health and mental health programs to support women who experience violence.

II.9

VIOLENCE IS A CONTAGIOUS DISEASE[6]

Gary Slutkin, M.D.
The University of Illinois at Chicago
Cure Violence (formerly CeaseFire)

Violence is a contagious disease. It meets the definitions of a disease and of being contagious—that is, violence is spread from one person to another. This paper will clarify (1) how violence is like infectious diseases historically by its natural history and by its behavior; (2) how violence specifically fits the basic infectious disease framework—and how we can use this framework to better understand what is known of the pathogenic processes of violence; and (3) how we can provide better guidance to future strategies for reducing violence, in order to get more predictable results, and develop a clearer path to putting violence into the past. This paper intends to clarify to the scientific and policy community, as well as the general public, how violence is acquired and biologically processed, and begins to outline how the spread of violence can be interrupted in short-term emergencies and longer term situations.

The Great Plagues and Violence

We begin by reminding ourselves that the great infectious diseases and violence have each killed tens to hundreds of millions of persons throughout history. Nothing else has caused this level of human fatalities. Yet, before we understood the causes of the great infectious diseases, that is, before discovering what was causing epidemics of leprosy, plague, tuberculosis, cholera, and other infectious diseases, we frequently treated the people affected as "bad people"; we blamed them for the problem, and in particular lamented their moral character. People with leprosy, plague, typhus, cholera, tuberculosis, and other maladies were frequently considered morally "bad," suffering stigma at a minimum, and in many cases worse treatment, including being put in dungeons, burnt at the stake, or thrown down wells.

Why did we do this?

We did this because we did not know—did not *yet* know—what was really happening. *Why* we did not know was because the causes and

---

[6] The author would like to acknowledge Charlie Ransford for his excellent technical help in the preparation of this manuscript; John Mills and David Heymann for their generous reviews of the infectious diseases sections; and Emile Bruneau and Jamil Zaki for their reviews of the neurobiology sections.

underlying processes were *invisible*. Plague, for example, is due to an invisible microorganism, carried by a flea, otherwise living inside a rat.

Who knew?

It was not until very recently in human history, the 17th century, that Anton Leuwenhoek, a tradesman and scientist-to-be, invented the microscope and discovered these previously invisible microorganisms (De Kruif, 1926). Another 200 years passed before Louis Pasteur, a chemist working as a consultant for the beer, wine, and milk industries who wanted to know why these products spoil, discovered that Leuwenhoek's organism *did something*. It was then up to Robert Koch to definitively prove that these invisible creatures caused animal and then human disease, first anthrax and then tuberculosis, the latter the most highly feared killer of the time (Green et al., 1982). These massively important discoveries built on each other and led over the course of the next few decades to the identification of most of the infectious organisms that cause epidemic diseases. This then led, over just a few short decades of human history that followed, to *entirely new and rational strategies* for reducing the amount and impact of these historical major killers—strategies as varied as case finding and therapy for tuberculosis; immunization for polio; and environmental sanitation, better food handling, the use of toilets, and hand washing for diarrheal disease (Dowling, 1977; Nelson and Williams, 2007; Heymann, 2008). One historic killer, smallpox, has been totally eliminated by a global immunization strategy. Some of these strategies, for example, using impregnated bed nets for malaria, are still evolving and improving.

But before these discoveries, and a new understanding of the problem, humankind was *stuck*.

Misdiagnosis and Mistreatment

It now seems as if the problem of violence, like the great infectious diseases of the past, has been stuck—not because we do not care enough, nor because we do not have enough money devoted to it, but because *we have made the wrong diagnosis*. Wrong diagnoses, in particular moralistic diagnoses, usually lead to ineffective and even *counterproductive* treatments and control strategies. Problems of mankind frequently do get stuck, sometimes for decades or even for the history of man, commonly because we do not correctly understand the problem *scientifically*, a step that is *required* to design and implement *rational and effective control measures*. It also seems that, historically, moralistic views and solutions usually fill that gap in understanding.

Moralistic ideas actually have a very poor record of solving problems, in part because people differ in their interpretations of moralistic ideas, and in part because they lack an understanding of the actual biology of the problem. Sometimes this is because of the fundamental attribution bias where we humans replace incomplete understanding with blame of others. As a result, people who have learned violence, as for those affected or infected with the great infectious diseases, have been misdiagnosed and mistreated. However, in 2012 we have more pieces of the puzzle. Violence can now be better understood scientifically, and as a result, there *must be a new strategy* to reduce and eliminate violence.

Scientific Understanding

Violence, for starters, is a phenomenon driven by the brain, as the brain regulates and controls behaviors. Like our previous lack of knowledge of infectious organisms, our knowledge of the invisible workings of the brain has also been a field in the dark (or dark ages). Recent discoveries, if brought together into a coherent framework, allow us to see that brain processes are in fact contagious too. If we can begin to draw on the fairly new research findings of social psychology (40 to 50 years old) and functional magnetic resonance imaging of the brain (15 to 20 years old), connect these findings with what is known from infectious disease epidemiology, and add the first studies of new therapeutic approaches—we can now define a new set of causations and strategies to *reduce violence more predictably.* Understanding epidemiology and invisible brain mechanisms will carry us farther out of the middle ages to new possibilities immediately available.

Infectious Diseases and Violence in Populations

There are three main characteristics of infectious diseases in *populations*: clustering, spread, and transmission. *Clustering* in space, or spatial grouping, is simple in concept and is characteristic of epidemic diseases. Clustering is shown in Figure II-1 for the infectious disease cholera in Bangladesh, and in Figure II-2 for violence in Chicago. *Spread* in epidemics is characteristically nonlinear. This may be one of the reasons why many researchers have difficulty attributing rises and falls to simple causative factors such as the economy or jobs. Nonlinear spread may occur as waves, frequently appearing as waves on top of waves. (This is characteristic of plague, smallpox, and many other infectious diseases; see Anderson and May, 1991, and as shown in Figure II-3 for the homicides in the United States over the past several decades.) This pattern of waves upon waves occurs because epidemics frequently consist of many epidemics, as spread itself diffuses and as contagious populations meet with new susceptible populations in new locations, and to be met with new provoking factors.

Another characteristic of spread in some circumstances is that seen from point source epidemics, sometimes exhibiting very rapid spread, as

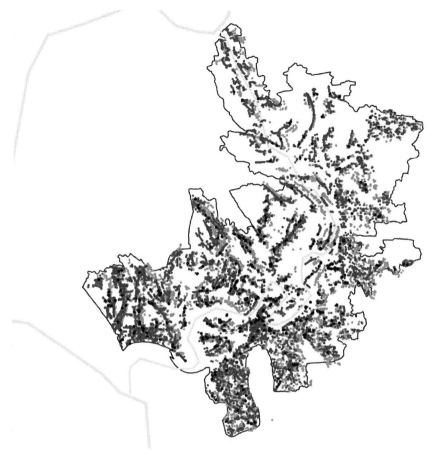

FIGURE II-1 Clustering in cholera epidemic, Bangladesh.
SOURCE: Ruiz-Moreno et al., 2010.

shown in Figures II-4 (cholera) and II-5 (violence). In these cases, one initial infectious event may cause many subsequent cases (for cholera, precipitated by an infected water source in Somalia; for the Rwanda genocide, the killing of the Rwandan president). Secondary epidemic waves are seen in each of these figures. With cholera, the secondary wave occurred when a new group of "susceptibles," in this case, refugees new to camp, became infected later. In Figure II-5, in this case, a violence/killing curve from Rwanda, the secondary wave similarly represents a new group of "*susceptibles*," in this case, persons who were previously hiding and then were found and killed (Verwimp, 2004). The similarities of these patterns reflect similar contagious dynamics.

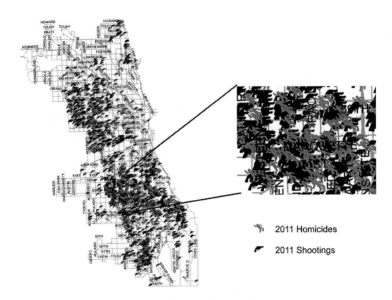

FIGURE II-2 Clustering in violence epidemic, Chicago.
NOTE: This data was provided by and belongs to the Chicago Police Department.
Any further use of this data must be approved by the Chicago Police Department.
Points of view or opinions contained within this document are those of the author
and do not necessarily represent the official position or policies of the Chicago
Police Department.
SOURCES: City of Chicago Data Portal.

Spread may be dramatic and rapid, or slow, depending on many factors. Rapid spread, well known for infectious diseases, is seen, for example,
in foodborne outbreaks, flu, or severe acute respiratory syndrome (SARS).
Rapid spread is seen in violence outbreaks such as gang wars, soccer riots,
or the Rwanda genocide. Dramatically rapid recent outbreaks include the
London and UK riots and even the "Arab Spring." Slower spread may be
seen in infectious disease outbreaks with longer incubation periods, such
as tuberculosis or AIDS—showing spread over decades—analogous to the
spread of violence in U.S. cities that showed increases over decades.

Some acute-phase outbreaks are from *common* or *point source transmission*, as described above; while longer term outbreaks are more commonly a result of *person-to-person transmission*. The speed of transmission
varies not only according to incubation periods of the infection, but also
according to the number of persons susceptible and infected from a given
source, as well as other factors. World War I was a violence outbreak
with multiple features including multiple "point sources" as new countries
"joined in." The result: 15 to 20 million persons died in less than 4.5 years.

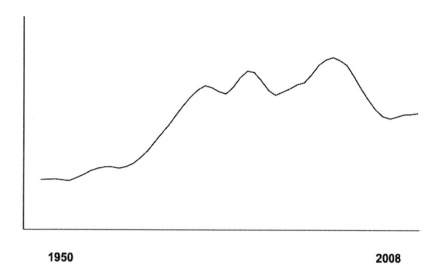

1950 **2008**

FIGURE II-3 Epidemic of killings in the United States, showing waves on top of waves.
SOURCES: BJS, 2005; FBI, 2008.

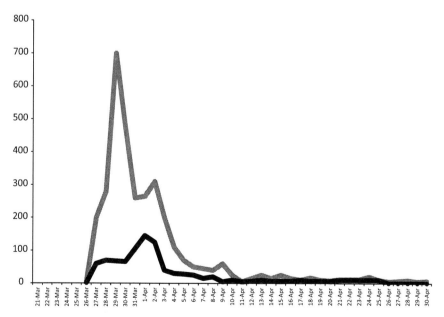

FIGURE II-4 Cholera—Gannet, Somalia.
SOURCE: Data from Farah, 1985, Figure 1.

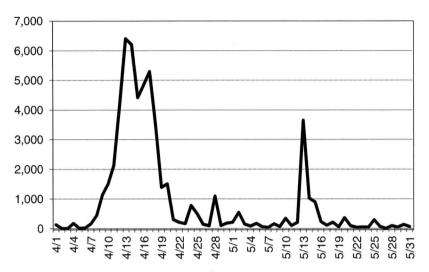

FIGURE II-5   Killings—Kibuya, Rwanda.
SOURCE: Data from Verwimp, 2004, Table 8.

    Transmission is the passage of an infection (or other condition) from one organism to another. The classic infectious diseases are transmitted by invisible infectious agents (e.g., viruses or bacteria), while violence is transmitted from human to human by equally invisible and now newly discovered pathways. Essentially transmission means that the disease or condition causes *something of itself* to be communicated, causing another person (or animal) to take on *some of the same characteristics*. In infectious disease language it means simply that being exposed to the disease makes it more likely that you will also develop the symptom complex characteristic of the same disease. This phenomenon has been shown for violence through many studies: people who are exposed to violence—either by observing, witnessing, or being subjected to violence themselves—are more likely to become what is called a perpetrator of violence (Widom, 1989; Stith et al., 2000; Reitzel-Jaffe and Wolfe, 2001; Ehrensaft et al., 2003; Guerra et al., 2003; Crooks et al., 2007; Huesmann and Kirwil, 2007; Kokko et al., 2009; Roberts et al., 2010). This is true for multiple forms of violence, as will be summarized and interpreted later in this paper.

Infectious Diseases and Violence in Individuals

    Violence not only shows the characteristics of infectious diseases in populations, but also the characteristics and key concepts of an infectious disease in an individual. These characteristics are listed in Table II-1 and

TABLE II-1   Concepts in Infectious Diseases in *Individuals*

Susceptibility (versus immunity, resistance)
Exposure, infectivity, transmission
Incubation, latency
Pathogenesis
Inapparent/subclinical
Carriers
Clinical spectrum (mild, severe, acute, intermittent, chronic)
Cure, relapse

shown schematically in Figure II-6. Space does not permit an in-depth review of these concepts, but the reader is referred to infectious disease textbooks (Anderson and May, 1991; Nelson and Williams, 2007). In brief, all of these concepts apply to violence, including susceptibility, exposure, transmission, incubation, and latency periods, as well as possibilities for different clinical courses and clinical outcomes, from minimal infection to death.

An infectious disease begins with *exposure* to the infection by a susceptible person. *Susceptibility* refers to the level (or lack) of *resistance* to infection for an individual; this could be due to the immune system (or other factors). For the usual infectious diseases, there are several mechanisms of immunity or resistance (e.g., mucosal cell integrity, or prior antibody or cell-mediated responses). Susceptibility and resistance are relative terms that can be overridden by dosage, types of exposure, or other circumstances. Drops in immunity can occur with time or context or due to changes in other biological or environmental circumstances, such as extreme temperatures or immune suppression. Immunity or resistance to exposure to violence may be a result of a family or peer environment in which views, behaviors, and norms against violence are very well established and maintained, and

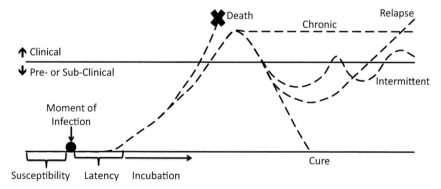

FIGURE II-6   Natural history of an infectious disease.

where alternative responses to exposure to violence are well supported, in particular among close peers (Berman et al., 1996; Osofsky, 1999; Garbino et al., 2002). In infectious disease language this is sometimes referred to as "herd immunity."

Incubation periods, defined as the time from infection to evidence of clinical disease, is variable in both infectious diseases and violence. In other words, influenza has an incubation period of days, while leprosy has incubation periods of years. The incubation period between HIV infection and AIDS can vary from months to decades. Some infectious diseases have extremely variable periods that can be weeks or years, for example, malaria or tuberculosis. Violence can also have quite varied incubation periods— rapid like cholera, such as for soccer riots, or gang wars, or the genocide in Rwanda (Verwimp, 2004), or longer incubation periods like tuberculosis, where the period between being subjected to child abuse and becoming a perpetrator of community or family violence may be years or decades later (Ehrensaft et al., 2003; Huesmann et al., 2003).

Even prolonged latencies of decades can be seen for both, where conditions for *reactivation* may be important (e.g., Huesmann et al., 2003). Interestingly both tuberculosis and violence show this ability for a person to be infected very young and then show active disease decades later. For example, a child younger than age 5 exposed to tuberculosis may show active disease in his late teens or early 20s; likewise, an abused child age 5 or less may exhibit violent behavior (community violence or be a child abuser himself) in the late teens, 20s, or later. The intervening years would be called the *incubation period* for an infectious disease, and could also be called an incubation period for violence.

Technically, whereas incubation period refers to the time to clinical disease, *latency* refers to time until infectivity to others. This infectivity or contagion can occur from among asymptomatic or presymptomatic persons, including carriers (see below), but also from persons who have not yet completed their incubation period, but who will become symptomatic later. Latency (or infectivity to others) can therefore come before or at the same time as the end of the incubation period; for example someone may spread a diarrheal infection before they are symptomatic. The violence analogy may be that persons may be provoking others to do violence, but do not (or yet) show the characteristic symptoms themselves (definition issues here will need to be worked out, such as whether persons who train others to do violence are showing a clinical syndrome or are just contagious to others).

Persons exposed to violence, as for infectious disease, can develop a *wide spectrum of possible clinical courses or outcomes* as a result of exposure, including no disease at all, a chronic or relapsing syndrome, disability, or death. *Carrier states* for infectious diseases include the classic example of "Typhoid Mary," a cook at the turn of the 20th century who was a carrier of Salmonella typhi (the bacterium causing typhoid fever), who although having no clinical disease herself was responsible for transmitting typhoid to more than 50 persons, with 3 deaths. The analogous situation for violence disease would be the person who causes others to become violent (e.g., through provocation) without manifesting overt violence disease themselves (all of these outcomes require treatment, in individual care and public health terms, once detected).

For each infectious agent, there are many different *clinical syndromes*. For example, with plague there are bubonic (lymphatic) and pneumonic (lung) syndromes. For tuberculosis the clinical picture may be that of respiratory disease, bone disease, or even meningitis. These may appear as different disease states, but they are in fact caused by the same microorganism or infection for each of these diseases mentioned.

Likewise there are different *violence* syndromes that are currently viewed as different "types of violence" to the general public, such as community violence, intimate partner violence, child abuse, and suicide. I suggest that these now be classified as *different syndromes of the same disease* because they derive from the same cause, but manifest under different circumstances. Differences in susceptibilities, contexts, and ages may play a part, just as polio may have different manifestations in very early ages than in childhood, or how influenza differentially affects older and very young persons.

Transmission: Including Transmission Across Syndromes

Exposure to violence increases the likelihood that the exposed person will commit violence, that is, to become a perpetrator (Kaufman and Zigler, 1987; Widom, 1989; Stith et al., 2000; Reitzel-Jaffe and Wolfe, 2001; Ehrensaft et al., 2003; Guerra et al., 2003; Crooks et al., 2007; Huesmann and Kirwil, 2007; Kokko et al., 2009; Roberts et al., 2010). In some cases the likelihood of being a victim may increase as well (Coid et al., 2001; Heyman and Slep, 2002; Ehrensaft et al., 2003). If we define *violence disease* as performing acts of physical harm to others or having acts performed against you, we can see through examining these different "categories" of violence that there is a *chain of transmission that occurs across syndromes*. By comparison, someone febrile and coughing with tuberculosis as well as someone with the disease in their lymph nodes or even brain (meningeal) tuberculosis are *all* infected with *M. tuberculosis*. We know that exposure to community violence can lead to perpetrating community violence (DuRant et al., 1994, 1996; Barkin et al., 2001; Kelly, 2010). In its most obvious example, the most likely predictor of a subsequent case of a shooting in street or gang violence is a previous shooting (Decker, 1996). Likewise, the greatest predictor of subsequent cases of colds, flu, SARS, Legionnaire's disease, and other infectious diseases is a prior case—and specifically exposure to a prior case—of that infection.

It has been said for a long time that violence begets violence, but it is *just as tuberculosis begets tuberculosis, or flu begets flu, that violence begets violence.*

We see violence causing violence in its most acute setting in cases of retaliations in gang violence (Decker, 1996) and even in war. For example, this was seen in what was called civil, or intrastate, wars, such as following the 2005 bombing of the Samarra Mosque in Iraq, or even what we call wars between states, or interstate wars, such as World War II. To an epidemiologist these should be known simply as violence outbreaks.

Furthermore, considerable evidence shows that having been a victim of violence increases the risk of someone perpetrating community violence (DuRant et al., 1994, 1996; Barkin et al., 2001; Morris et al., 2002; Mullins et al., 2004; Kelly, 2010). However, it is also now clear that exposure to *community* violence (outside the family unit) leads to an increased likelihood of *family* violence, both against intimate partners and abuse of (or violence against) children, as well as an increased risk of violence *against self* or suicide (Mullins et al., 2004; Devries et al., 2011). Furthermore, exposure to (observing) violence between parents leads to a greater likelihood of being a perpetrator of intimate partner violence (Stith et al., 2000; Reitzel-Jaffe and Wolfe, 2001; Ehrensaft et al., 2003; Naved and Persson, 2005) or child abuse (Kaufman and Zigler, 1987; Heyman and Slep, 2002; Milner et al., 2010), and to being exposed to community violence (Hanson et al., 2006). Being traumatized as a victim of *child abuse* also leads to *community violence* (Widon, 1989; Crooks et al., 2007), intimate partner violence (Stith et al., 2000; Ehrensaft et al., 2003), and child abuse (Kaufman and Zigler, 1987; Heyman and Slep, 2002; Milner et al., 2010). Exposure to war and political violence, particularly when accompanied by posttraumatic stress disorder, leads to being a perpetrator of intimate partner violence and community violence (Archer and Gartner, 1976; Landau and Pfeffermann, 1988; Sela-Shayovitz, 2005; Catani et al., 2008; Clark et al., 2010; Landau et al., 2010; Teten et al., 2010; Widome et al., 2011). Exposure to violence in the media leads to the perpetration of violence in the community and at home (Huesmann et al., 2003), as does witnessing violence in video games (Huesmann, 2010). Suicide, a type of violence directed at oneself, can also frequently follow exposure to intimate partner violence, community violence, (Cavanaugh et al., 2011; Devries et al., 2011) or other suicides (Gould, 2001; Gould et al., 2003; Jeong et al., 2012).

Further evidence of this *cross-syndrome connection* has been shown, for example, in studies by Eric Dubow and Rowell Huesmann in war settings. These studies have shown, in the setting of Israeli Jew, Israeli Arab, or Palestinian Arab, that exposure to or involvement in ethnopolitical violence leads to the performance of violence against spouses and peers, removing any pretense of the primacy of "reasons" for violence (Dubow et al., 2009; Landau et al., 2010). Like the example of different forms of tuberculosis, something common has been transmitted—in this case, a tendency toward violence, likely mediated by underlying biological processes. A violence disease or predisease state is present.

Therefore, something is being transmitted across and between various "types" of violence. Because something common is being transmitted, likely involving common intermediate brain pathways, these different "types" of violence should be called syndromes of the same *violence disease.*

Definitions—Violence Is a Contagious Disease— and Is Like an Infectious Disease

Disease

Dorland's Illustrated Medical Dictionary, 32nd Edition (2010), defines a disease as "any deviation or interruption of structure or function of a part, organ, or system of the body, as manifested by *characteristic symptoms and signs* (causing morbidity and mortality); the etiology, pathology, and prognosis may be known or unknown." The classic Oxford dictionary defines a disease as a "*pathological condition* of a part, organ, or system of an organism resulting from various causes, such as infection, genetic defect, or environmental stress, and characterized by an *identifiable group of signs or symptoms.*"[7]

I would suggest that the characteristic signs and symptoms of violence are the behavioral actions that cause or attempt to cause physical injury to another person or to one's self, and that these constitute a disease. I would add that anyone who has suffered physical injury as a result of violence, and in some cases been traumatically threatened, may also be considered infected, or diseased. In other words I am suggesting that both what is called perpetrator and what is called victim in the current literature be considered as *violence infected* or having the violence disease. I also suggest that, until we develop a clear marker for infection, we consider most persons that are exposed as infected, and clinical disease as the presence of symptoms. In

---

[7] A second definition, referring to a condition of society, reads "a condition or tendency, as of society, regarded as abnormal and harmful."

many infectious diseases, there are many more people infected than have clinical disease.

Contagious and Infectious

Dorland's medical dictionary defines contagious as "capable of being transmitted from one individual to another; communicable." This has been shown in the preceding section of this paper, for many clinical syndromes of violence. Violence is a contagious disease.

For infectious disease, some definitions or medical experts may prefer or choose to require a free-living microorganism, or physical agent, and for them violence may not be considered an infectious disease. However, not all microorganisms or microscopically transmissible definable entities are free living, for example, viruses or prions. Some medical textbooks refer to infectious as having a presence of a microorganism, but not always (Dorland, 2010; Stedman, 2012). The characteristic of infectivity itself is frequently synonymous with contagious or communicable, and this sometimes differential in medical textbooks may be simply conforming to the need for practitioners to be able to use antimicrobial agents or conventional medical approaches. However, as a practitioner, I am aware of the existence of many infectious diseases in which we do not have effective antimicrobial agents nor immunization (e.g., Ebola, Marburg, many viral diseases, antibiotic-resistant diseases, and for many years, AIDS), yet we still need to have effective approaches.

Using the term *contagious* remains technically sound, while avoiding possible controversies around the need for a physical agent that the term *infectious* might require for some.

Means of Transmission

Infectious diseases have many routes and means of transmission, from respiratory to fecal-oral to bloodborne to vectorborne. A full listing is available in most infectious disease textbooks. Pathogens can enter via the respiratory tract, gut, skin, or other routes to then cause dysfunction or dysregulation of one or more organs.

In the case of violence, we are looking at a process clearly mediated by the brain, with transmission appearing to come from at least two possible pathways: visual observation (o) and direct victimization (v). A third mechanism may be considered intentional training (t), for example by the military. Following transmission there are mediating factors that help predict the likelihood of a "take," and intervening or mediating mechanisms facilitate whether exposure or infection is likely to result in disease, which in this case is a violent act.

Mechanisms of Contagion or Infectivity, and Pathogenesis of Disease Formation

Biological mechanisms underlie the acquisition of infectious and other diseases. These are not just mechanisms of destruction or tissue damage, but frequently changes in organ *function* such as regulation, or dysregulation (e.g., immune responses in the lung to tuberculosis, flu or cold viruses).

For infectious processes, biological mechanisms must be elucidated for acquisition, and pathogenesis and mediators of progression defined. With respect to violence, where the behavior is being transmitted, Albert Bandura showed that social learning or what we could call imitating or modeling, is a principal mechanism for the acquisition of behaviors (Bandura and Huston, 1961; Bandura et al., 1961; Bandura, 1977, 1986). Several variables cause behaviors to more likely be copied, such as proximity to the learner and dose, effectively the amount, or intensity of exposure. The biological mechanisms here are not well known, but may involve cortical mirror-type of circuits, which are likely more complicated than mirror neurons alone (Iacoboni et al., 2005; Uddin et al., 2007). Besides acquiring simple behaviors, there is evidence for the acquisition of "scripts" or more likely responses to common events (Huesmann and Eron, 1984; Huesmann and Kirwil, 2007). Such behaviors are then maintained in large part by how the brain maintains habits, and by the largely invisible force of social pressure or expectations of peers. It may be that rewards for social approval, or other cues to belonging to social networks (e.g., positive reputation, consensus) may be mediated by dopamine-like reward pathways (Baumeister and Leary, 1995; Izuma et al., 2008; Losin et al., 2012). Perhaps equally importantly, it appears that *not* belonging (or social isolation) engages the same brain regions (shows up on brain scans) with some of the same patterns as physical pain (Panksepp, 1998; Eisenberger and Lieberman, 2004, 2005; Macdonald and Leary, 2005; Eisenberger, 2011, 2012), and is therefore avoided at great cost. Additional research shows that trauma (an outcome of exposure to violence) causes dysregulation in the limbic system and prefrontal cortex leading to hypervigilance (Margolin and Gordis, 2000; Perry, 2001; Fonzo et al., 2010), and hostile attribution (Joshi and O'Donnell, 2003) to perceived insults, resulting in more rapid and less regulated responses to real or perceived insults. These regions are affected by exposure to violence (Wang et al., 2009; Hummer et al., 2010). These mechanisms appear to be some of those that may underlie the infectivity of violence itself, as well as those underlying the capabilities for escalation, and rapid recruitment of individuals and further events.

In other words, both the infectious nature of the violence disease and the intervening brain processes causing the violence disease process can, at least in part, be defined, or at least speculated on, with refinements and new research certain to continue. These pathways could be considered, for example, parallel to how infection by the cholera bacterium causes the severe diarrhea characteristic of cholera disease, not by *destroying* the intestines, but by causing a *dysregulation* of salt and water transport in the intestine (with V. cholera, the dysregulation is manifested by a blocking of the Na-K pump that absorbs water in the small intestine, thereby causing diarrhea and likewise the perpetuation and additional infectivity to others of the clinical syndrome). Similarly, brain processes affected by observation and trauma cause both *alterations and dysregulation* of specific mechanisms and pathways in the brain noted above.

It is important to add that not all people infected with infectious diseases (or violence) will show disease. In fact for many infectious diseases, a minority of persons develop clinical disease following infection. For example, approximately 2 billion people in the world are currently infected with tuberculosis, but only approximately 9 million have cases of the clinical disease, with 1.4 million deaths per year (WHO, 2012). Many factors influence the likelihood of disease, and both infectious diseases and violence are more likely to "take" and progress with larger doses, particular contexts, less immunity, certain types of exposures, and absent or ineffective treatment.

Treating Violence as an Infectious Epidemic Is Effective

Three main strategies are used in reversing infectious epidemic processes. These are (1) detecting and interrupting ongoing and potentially new infectious events; (2) determining who are most likely to cause further infectious events from the infected population and then reducing their likelihood of developing disease and/or subsequently transmitting; and (3) changing the underlying social and behavioral norms, or environmental conditions, that directly relate to the spread of the infection (Nelson and Williams, 2007; Heymann, 2008).

The Cure Violence (previously known as CeaseFire Health) Method uses these same principles that are used to reverse infectious epidemics to prevent and reverse epidemic violence. The Cure Violence Method is therefore, both a science and community/street-based intervention. The method was designed in the late 1990s in Chicago, piloted in 2000 in West Garfield Park, replicated in multiple cities throughout the United States and other countries, independently evaluated, and is now considered a best practice by several national and international organizations and publications (DOJ, 2009; *The Economist*, 2009; Skogan et al., 2009; U.S. Conference of Mayors, 2012; Webster et al., 2012).

The Cure Violence Method begins by analyzing the clusters involved and transmission dynamics, and uses several new categories of disease control workers—including violence interrupters, outreach behavior change agents, and community coordinators—to interrupt transmission (or the contagion) to stop the spread of the violence disease and to change underlying norms. Workers are trained as disease control workers, similar to tuberculosis or HIV/AIDS workers or those looking for first cases of bird flu or SARS (Slutkin et al., 2006; Ransford, in press).

Tuberculosis workers help find cases and ensure that persons are sufficiently rendered noninfectious, albeit in the case of tuberculosis it is through the use of antimicrobial agents. However, tuberculosis outreach workers also require the use of persuasion (e.g., for taking medications) to ensure that effective change is occurring. Cure Violence disease control workers have training in modern methods of persuasion, behavior change, and changing community norms—all essential for limiting spread of outbreaks of violence. The principles underpinning the approach come from modern knowledge of social psychology and brain research, just as the principles of controlling other infectious disease flow from understanding their underlying mechanisms and patterns of flow.

Some of these principles include using persons from the same "in-group," which causes less defiance and more trust, credibility, and access. A number of cognitive processes are sensitive to group membership and for assessing "us" or "them" (Mathur et al., 2010; Bruneau et al., 2012), and determining whether someone is working in your own interest or not. The modern practice of behavior change requires the use of credible messengers, as well as ensuring that the new behaviors are acceptable and feel right socially, including being able to overcome social, physical, and other barriers (for example, the pressure that other groups are doing it). Messages need to be constructed to include new information about the behavior and new skills practiced along with developing opportunities for positive peer reactions and avoiding negative peer reactions. Violence interrupters' training also includes new and newly anticipated responses so that new brain circuits can be used in the short and longer term, as well as new social pressure and direction for "belonging."

Changing norms is done most effectively by putting some of these practices in play to scale as well as questioning existing norms and proscribing new norms at population levels. As thoughts, behavioral scripts, and norms are transmissible, new scripts and norms are developed and a new set of behaviors becomes more normal. Interruption is essential; however, brain processes, including preexisting emotional dysregulation as well as continued peer pressures to belong, remain problems if unattended to or untreated.

Changing norms is done most effectively by putting some of these new practices into play to scale—by developing a cascading diffusion through social networks, gradually accumulating the new responses. This is accelerated by systematically questioning existing norms and proscribing new norms at population levels. As thoughts, behavioral scripts, and norms are transmissible, new scripts and norms are developed and a new set of behaviors becomes more normal. Interruption remains essential; as brain processes, including preexisting emotional dysregulation difficulties—as well as continued peer pressures to belong—remain problems if unattended to or untreated.

These methods have resulted in reductions in shootings and killings of 16 to 28 percent directly attributed to the strategy by time series analysis (see Table II-2); from 41 to 73 percent overall (Skogan et al., 2009); and in its first outside replication, in Baltimore, reduced shootings and killings by 34 to 56 percent (Webster et al., 2012). The initial implementation has been replicated in more than 20 communities in Baltimore, Chicago, New York, and several other cities with large reductions in violence found by independently performed studies commissioned by the U.S. Department of Justice, the Centers for Disease Control and Prevention, and Johns Hopkins University (Skogan et al., 2009; Webster et al., 2012).

This new approach is now being used by more than a dozen U.S. cities and a growing number of countries, including in Kenya to prevent or reduce election violence, South Africa to reduce and prevent community violence, and Iraq to reduce and prevent interpersonal and intertribal violence.

The idea of violence as a contagious or infectious disease is rapidly catching hold. In 2008, the *New York Times Sunday Magazine* cover story by Alex Kotlowitz about the Cure Violence epidemic control method (formerly referred to as CeaseFire) ran with the title "Is Urban Violence a

TABLE II-2 National Institute of Justice External Evaluation of CeaseFire Chicago: Three Approaches to Impact Analysis

	Change in Violence Due to Program		
	Shootings Down	Hot Spots Cooler[a]	Retaliation Homicides Down
Auburn–Gresham	−16%/−21%	−15%	−100%
East Garfield Park	Not evaluated		−100%
Englewood			−100%
Logan Square	−21%		−100%
Rogers Park		−40%	No change
Southwest	−20%/−23%		−100%
West Garfield Park	−22%/−28%	−24%	−46%
West Humboldt Park		−17%	−50%

[a] Hot spots are locations where shootings are particularly concentrated. Cooling indicates a reduction in this concentration after implementation.

Virus?" The 2009 *Economist* special "World in 2009 Edition" described the epidemic control approach and predicted that this would be "the approach that would come to prominence." The recent award-winning documentary *The Interrupters* also highlighted the disease control approach.

The science, and the public understanding that follows this science, are bringing us into a new era. This new era is an era of *discovery*—but more importantly of *transition*. We can now leave the days of a vocabulary of "bad people" and "enemies" and apply a scientific understanding and a scientific approach to this problem. Violence has all of the historical, population, and individual characteristics of an infectious disease. It has routes of transmission, incubation periods, and different clinical syndromes and outcomes. There are definable biological processes underlying the pathogenesis. In addition, treatment as an infectious disease is effective. All of this requires more refinement and research. We are still performing research and refining our approach with tuberculosis, cholera, and malaria as well, but at least we have taken these problems out of the moral, medieval, and superstitious realms of evil and dungeons.

The advantages to this new and scientific understanding and approach to violence are countless. We can more proactively *avoid exposure* and develop new ways of responding to exposure. We can treat and develop *better methods of treating* infected persons and communities. We can further strengthen the Cure Violence and other early epidemic control approaches referred to here. Most of all, we can now move away from counterproductive practices into the *modern era*.

Violence is a contagious disease. This is good news as this knowledge offers new strategies for control. There are massive implications for how to better treat urban violence, as well as for international conflicts. As we have done before—for plague, typhus, leprosy, and so many other diseases—we can now apply *science-based strategies* and, as we did for the great infectious diseases, similarly move violence into the past.

II.10

EMOTIONAL AND EVOLUTIONARY ASPECTS OF CONTAGIOUS VIOLENCE: OVERLAPPING FACTORS IN THE GENESIS OF DIVERSE TYPES OF NON-SANCTIONED HUMAN AGGRESSION[8]

Jeffrey Victoroff, M.D.
University of Southern California Keck School of Medicine

The Evolution and Mechanism of Aggression

Animals employ aggression in many ways to serve many intermediate goals, such as acquisition of nutrients, defense against predators, social control, and sexual success. However, the reason that aggressive behavior occurs throughout the kingdom Animalia is simply that natural selection favors the genetic replication of individuals who are more likely to survive and reproduce, and aggression facilitates inclusive fitness in multiple ways.

Some aggression is collective. For example, social insects such as ants and bees act aggressive collectively to advance and protect their fitness interests (Moffett, 2011). Social primates such as chimpanzees or spider monkeys coordinate their aggression in ways that enhance individual and (indirectly) group benefit (Mitani et al., 2010). Other social primates such as humans routinely engage in collective aggression. Examples include cooperative hunting, intergroup raiding and defense, police-like social control, and later in history, the emergence of specialization of subgroups who participate more than other community members in warfare. This type of collective aggression seems to have evolved, at least in part, because reciprocal altruism requires and rewards a costly signal demonstrating risk taking on behalf of the in-group (Barclay and Willer, 2007; Miller, 2007). Evidence shows that the very existence of human civilization derives from the innovation of such pro-social collective aggression (Bowles, 2009). Soldiers join armies and wage wars to demonstrate their commitment to reciprocal altruism. Genetic variants and cultural trends that tended to perpetuate or enhance such aggression have been favored, perhaps for millions of years of hominine evolution. It is possible, but remains to be shown that the success of Cro Magnons over Neanderthals was strongly related to this early modern human trait.

The human brain embodies aggressive potential. Multiple anatomical regions play complex interactive roles in mediating individual or collective aggression, including (1) brainstem (which help to monitor the environment, mediate arousal, and regulate the many neurotransmitters and neurohumoral agents that either increase or permit aggression); (2) the

---

[8] The author wishes to gratefully acknowledge Janice Adelman, Ph.D., for her valuable contribution to the analysis of the data on Palestinian terror attacks and their support.

hypothalamus (which helps regulate multiple steroid and peptide hormones relevant to the mediation and moderation of aggression, such as serotonin, dopamine, cortisol, and the nonapeptides—arginine vasopressin and oxytocin); (3) the medial temporal lobar allocortex, especially the amygdala, which plays an important role in both detecting and learning threat; and (4) the cingulate gyrus (which mediates drive or motivation, as well as integrating cortical/liminal activity with subcortical/subliminal activity); and several regions of the neocortex (e.g., the dorsolateral prefrontal cortex, which mediates conscious or semiconscious decision making, and the ventromedial prefrontal cortex, which plays multiple roles, including assessment of social circumstances and inhibition of impulsivity) (Adams, 2006; Victoroff et al., 2011; Comai et al., 2012). Differences occur in the level of aggressiveness of individuals who are not accounted for by focal brain anatomy, but correlate instead with a variety of genetic polymorphisms that appear to underlie brain function, or with physiological variations such as hormone levels, central electrophysiology, or autonomic nervous system function.

Therefore, an innate capacity for and tendency toward aggressive behavior, embodied in the brain, represents an important and valuable outcome of the coevolution of genes and cultures.

For better or for worse—and perhaps contrary to the conventions of intuition—the same evolutionary, cultural, and neurobiological factors endow humans with a capacity for antisocial aggression, whether perpetrated by individuals or groups. More aggressive individuals, even psychopathic individuals, are merely expressing one perfectly adaptive life history option for maximizing fitness: the live-fast-die-young strategy (Wolf et al., 2007; Victoroff et al., 2011). Examples of this adaptive strategy include the commission of unsanctioned murder, rape, and participation in violent juvenile gang activity, and participation in violent adult organized criminal activity.

Individual and collective aggression varies. Some individuals and some groups indisputably exhibit relatively higher or lower frequencies and severities of individual (e.g., homicide) or collective (e.g., gang-related homicide) antisocial aggression. At least eight overarching factors contribute to the variation in observed aggressive behavior over time and space:

1. Individual genetic and epigenetic variation, for example, proaggressive polymorphisms such as the short allelic variant of the gene for monoaminoxidase, the A1 allele of the dopamine receptor D2 gene, the short variation of a repetitive sequence in the transcriptional control region of the serotonin (5-HT) transporter gene (SCL6A4, 5-HTT), or shorter repeat length of androgen receptor gene CAG.
2. Individual congenital/infancy factors, such as pre- or perinatal injury, fetal exposure to neurotoxins, birth complications, infantile illness, or larger body size at birth.

3. Individual variations in biological endophenotypes such as atypical neurotransmitter levels, transmission dynamics, cytokine levels, neuroendocrine traits and states associated with both steroid and peptide hormone levels, atypical central electrophysiology, atypical amygdalar responsiveness, atypical autonomic nervous system function, or a recently hypothesized reward deficiency syndrome linked to atypical monoamine function.

4. Individual postnatal environmental factors, such maternal deprivation, child abuse or harsh punishment, neurotoxicity (e.g., lead paint exposure), anabolic steroid exposure, prescribed agents, or substance abuse (note that a distinction is made between the *comorbidity* of substance abuse and aggression, described below, and the occurrence of aggression-promoting *neurotoxicity* due to substance abuse), stressful events or losses (with or without posttraumatic stress disorder or PTSD), exposure to media incitement or modeling, head trauma, or, rarely, infectious disease.

5. Occurrence of significant Axis I or Axis II mental disorders, including conduct disorder, schizophrenia, autism, antisocial personality disorders, borderline personality disorder, mood disorders, PTSD, dissociative disorders, substance abuse, posttraumatic encephalopathy, and combinations of such disorders, especially comorbid thought disorder and substance abuse.

6. Variation in personality traits, including callous-unemotional traits, impulsivity, antisocial traits, sensation seeking or risk taking, seeking or defense of dominance, fearlessness, or low frustration tolerance.

7. Variations in cognitive style or intellectual capacity, including the occurrence of learning disabilities or attention deficit disorders.

8. Group environmental factors, such as cultural tolerance or support of violent problem solving or revenge killings, socioeconomic factors reducing the availability of alternate life history strategies such as marriage and/or gainful employment, social learning of aggression, and social network factors exposing individuals to other innovators from whom they learn the efficacy of aggression. Such group factors inspire the coalescence of like-minded persons into groups sharing an identity. This dynamic transcends ideology and drives collective aggression of multiple types. For example, as Crenshaw opined (1986, p. 395):

> Terrorist organizations become countercultures, with their own values and norms, into which new groups are indoctrinated. . . . They are in this respect similar to youth gangs or nonpolitical cults and sects.

Indeed, evidence suggests that while individuals with some genomes may be inherently at lower or higher risk of phenotypic aggression, and that certain environmental exposures increase the risk of adopting a violent lifestyle, it is most likely that aggressiveness is determined by *bidirectional interactions* between genes, epigenetic variations, endophenotypes, and environmental exposures (Veenema, 2009; Cohen, 2010; Nordstrom et al., 2011). For example, a child born with a neurobiologically based reward-deficiency syndrome may both be attracted to risk-taking behaviors and to substances of abuse. Seeking rewarding substances will not only plunge that child into a problematic social milieu, but may produce brain damage that will exacerbate his or her antisocial traits. A child who experiences early stress may develop the endophenotype of altered neuropeptide function, causing a lowered threshold for reactive aggression (Fries et al., 2005). Similarly, a child born with a suboptimal central processing system for emotional regulation may be more vulnerable to early victimization (Rudolph et al., 2011)—a known precursor of gang participation.

In essence, variations in cognitive style and emotional reactivity based on evolutionary diversity of adaptive life history strategies lead to variations in expression of both individual and, perhaps, collective aggression.

The Useful Metaphor of Contagion

Curiously, however, despite decades of research, variation in the rate of individual and collective aggression cannot be completely accounted for by factors that intuitively would explain the waxing and waning in violence. Neither economic markers, group humiliation nor dispossession, availability of weapons, exposure to psychotropic substances, nor any other plausible factors have been shown to account for all of the up and down swings in the rate of communal violence (Gilligan, 1997; Zimring and Hawkins, 1997; Fagan et al., 1998; Rutter et al., 1998).

This observation has perhaps been the inspiration for a number of novel theories about the ultimate genesis of criminal violence, including the hypothesis that violence is contagious. That is, entirely apart from changes in age distribution, population frequency of proaggressive genetic polymorphisms, rates of child abuse, rates of poverty, or political oppression, scholars have noted what appears to be a cyclical pattern of the occurrence of community violence and have proposed that the spreads and contractions in the rate of such violence may represent a phenomenon that is strongly analogous to the spreads and contractions in the occurrence of infectious diseases.

An abundant literature has emerged over the past 60 years examining the plausibility that the concept of contagion usefully accounts for trends in a wide variety of social phenomenon. Contagious diffusion—or innovation

followed by imitation—has been proposed as an important cause of biobehavioral trends as diverse as medical innovation, sexual behaviors, team
behavior, mood, entry into first marriage, smoking, teenage suicide, and
even everyday decision making.

Many forms of political aggression have also been attributed to contagion, including political unrest, political coups, civil wars, riots, ethnoreligious conflict, and terrorism (Bandura, 1973; Huff and Lutz, 1974; Li and
Thompson, 1975; Bohstedt, 1994; Fox, 2004; Sedgwick, 2007; Nacos,
2009; Kathman, 2011). More specifically with regard to the waxing and
waning of community violence, multiple authors have offered theoretical
and empirical reasons to believe that such violence spreads in a contagious
manner (Fagan and Davies, 2004; Patten and Arboleda-Florez, 2004; Fagan
et al., 2007; Papachristos, 2009).

According to this hypothesis, individuals innovatively adapt their behavior to the goals and circumstances. Some will be innovators of violence.
As other people observe the innovators, especially if the innovators are
seen to achieve important life goals, imitation will occur (e.g., Fagan et
al., 2007). Bandura (1973, p. 215) described the dynamics of this clearly:

> Social contagion of new styles and tactics of aggression conforms to a
> pattern that characterizes the transitory changes of most other types of
> collective activities: New behavior is initiated by a salient example; it
> spreads rapidly in a contagious fashion; after it has been widely adopted,
> it is discarded.

(If those societies ever discard interpersonal and intergroup violence as a
behavioral tactic.)

Authorities in quantitative sociology have proposed that, in such cases
of contagious diffusion of behavior, independent of external factors one
would expect phenomena such as the level of community violence to vary
in a cyclical pattern that will roughly approximate a sigmoid curve. Yet
the inevitability of historic or demographic factors playing a role has led
to the prediction that that curve would be *asymmetric*. Indeed, Fagan and
colleagues (2007) published evidence of just such a curve describing the
otherwise inexplicable waxing and waning of handgun violence in New
York City between 1968 and 2000 (see Figure II-7).

Figure II-7 from Fagan et al. (2007) may be compared with our preliminary analysis of data from the Israeli/Palestinian conflict. With Janice Adelman, I recently analyzed both the occurrence of terrorist attacks and the
level of Palestinian community support expressed for such attacks between
January 1996 and January 2011. Our initial hypothesis was that, in accordance with Crenshaw's admonition (1986, 1995) that the behavior of terror
groups is often (but not always) linked to social approval and communal
support for that behavior, and her comment that this is particularly the case

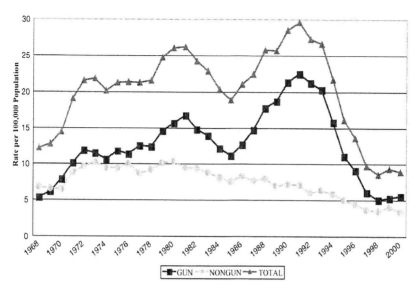

FIGURE II-7 Gun and nongun homicide rates per 100,000 persons, 1968-2000, New York City.
SOURCE: Fagan et al., 2007; used by permission.

with regard to Hamas (Crenshaw, 2000), one would observe a time-lagged correlation between measures of communal support and measures of militant action, with attacks increasing as support for those attacks increased. We also speculated that major historical events, such as Ariel Sharon's stepping onto the Temple Mount and the construction of the security wall, would perturb the relationship between communal support and attacks. The data were more complex. While some upswings or downswings in attacks seemed explicable by reference to communal support or major historical/policy changes, an asymmetric quasi-sigmoid curve emerged that could not be accounted for entirely by these factors (see Figure II-8).

Comparing Figures II-7 and II-8, and acknowledging the major differences in the types of aggression and the methodology of data acquisition, one is at least tempted to consider the possibility that (a) contagion-like dissemination of aggressive behaviors may help to explain otherwise mysterious fluctuations, and (b) the early prediction of asymmetric quasi-sigmoid trajectories in the occurrence of such phenomena seems defensible.

Obviously, if there exists an asymmetric sigmoidal trend in the occurrence of communal violence of widely disparate types, that pattern of variation-with-time has a cause. For both theoretical reasons and because of our Palestinian data, I propose a hybrid model of the contagion hypothesis.

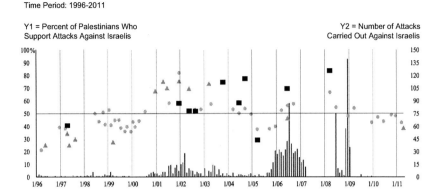

FIGURE II-8　Plot of support for attacks (Y1) and number of perpetrated attacks (Y2) over time.
SOURCE: Victoroff and Adelman, 2012.

Violence waxes and wanes *in part* because of innovation and imitation. Yet it is vital to acknowledge the multiplicity of other factors that may contribute to or cause major changes in community rates of individual or collective violence. Innumerable such factors have been proposed or identified—from the population density of proaggressive genetic polymorphisms, to the occurrence of harsh discipline or parental abuse, to the rate of childhood heavy metal neurotoxicity, to the cohesiveness of the community, and to the structural stresses of deprivation and income inequality.

The neurobiological mechanisms by which these factors influence the central nervous systems of participants in violence are slowly being elucidated. At this point, it is premature to propose a weighting of factors or tight localization of systems, circuits, neurons, and neurohumors contributing to the causal pathway. Yet one conclusion has become inescapable: People do not simply choose to become violent by the rational exercise of free will.

That is, according to the discipline of behavioral economics, all decisions are rational. Humans are assumed to have evolved rational decision-making nervous systems, and indeed, the primate brain appears to contain systems that internally represent values, calculate risks and benefits, and make useful behavioral choices.

But classical microeconomic algorithms fail to provide accurate predictions of real human decision making for several reasons. First, contrary to a basic assumption of rational choice theory, empirical evidence shows that humans are not good intuitive calculators of risk and benefit. Second, there is considerable individual variation in human decision making, mediated not only by biases such as risk aversion, ambiguity aversion, and choice blindness, but by variations in numeracy—all neural operations potentially subject to genetic and epigenetic variation. Both intra- and interindividual variation occurs in emotional biasing of decisions. Emotional framing, for instance, makes brains process moral options with different tissue and outcomes. Innate and acquired variation may alter decision calculus. Fourth, recent research has identified systematic cultural-bound differences in punishment decisions. These recent findings may be especially relevant to the analysis of Islamist extremist behaviors; compared with most Westerners, those in some Middle Eastern societies appear more willing to engage in costly and irrational "antisocial punishment," which may take the form of vengeance even when such actions are self-defeating.

All these real-world violations of economic prediction are sometimes excused as so-called bounded rationality—the claim that hominids simply lack the calculating capacity for reliable self-interested choice (Simon, 1955). It is possible that one major conceptual error underlying the misguided enthusiasm for rational choice models is the untenable assumption that human brains are serial processors (Simon, 1967). Although some authorities cling to the framework of quantitative predictive validity by calling their new calculus "neuroeconomics," far too many deviations from rational economic predictions have been observed to sustain a hypothesis that economic balancing of expected risks and benefits plays a major role in the occurrence of most human actions. Newer models of decision making at least acknowledge an element of random or stochastic choice that only slowly drifts toward reward maximization (Soltani et al., 2006). Revising the rational choice/econometric theories of the past, a new generation of scholars is exploring the interaction between emotions and decision making.

The deep philosophical issue that lurks beneath these investigations is the popular assumption of free will. That issue cannot be addressed adequately in this brief essay. Suffice it to say that, from the biologist's perspective, the evidence for human free will is just as robust as the evidence for precognition. The illusion of free will is perhaps best regarded as a curious adaptation, perhaps confined to species with cortices, the value of which remains to be elucidated.

Still, rather than considering the overwhelming evidence of rationality violations as debunking a myth of rational man, I propose that such discoveries open the door to refinements that will lead to a better, wiser, biologically informed psychoneuroeconomics. Human actions on this earth are determined by actions in brains. Actions in brains are determined by physical laws, the investigation of which remains in its early infancy. That incipient science is beginning to attend far more to the importance of emotions. Emotions are central to determining who among us ultimately acts violently and who deals with life's challenges without resort to violence.

Emotions are subjective feelings in response to either internal or external stimuli. They derive both from innate, inborn, and probably genitivally and epigenetically determined personality traits and from many fetal, childhood, and later developmental and environmental influences. When one of three boys in a family joins a gang and the others do not, it is insufficient to point to political structural factors, economic factors, or even parenting as the trigger. The gang joiner is different. He or she probably exhibits different types and degrees of emotional and physiological responsiveness to loss, to perceived threat, to perceived injustice, to out-group exposure, and to the rewards of peer acceptance. I predict that empirical research will identify both emotional and biological traits that distinguish gang participants from the nonparticipant siblings.

Discoveries in this domain potentially have implications for the prevention of violence. If, for example, early childhood depression or traumatic brain injury were shown to account for a significant amount of the variance in gang participation, the community could redouble its efforts to provide comprehensive maternal health care, and to protect young brains from injury (e.g., by evidence-based revisions in return to play guidelines in youth sports).

Cause(s) of Violence

Based on the foregoing discussion, it becomes clear why any unidisciplinary approach to the terrible dilemma of nonsanctioned human violence will founder. The metaphor of contagion (which shares a great deal of its empirical authority with findings from studies of network theory), may help to account for some aspects of trends in violence over time. Yet, rather than searching for "the" cause of a violent event, it may be useful to consider the interaction of multiple causes.

The epidemiology of primary injury prevention also offers a potentially useful way to conceptualize this kind of causality: the Haddon Matrix. Haddon matrixes were originally devised by physician William Haddon as a new way to analyze the causes of injuries and the multiple potential avenues for prevention. This framework alerts policy makers that factors influencing injuries—including violent injuries—are subject to the influence of three overlapping tiers of potential intervention: individual behavioral, environmental, and public policy. Since Haddon's introduction of this conceptual framework, it has been applied to diverse forms of injury, including

- tiger escapes,
- crocodile attacks,
- burns,
- amusement park accidents,
- chemical warfare terrorism,
- the 2005 London bombings,
- workplace violence, and
- youth gun violence.

For purposes of illustration, I have prepared two preliminary Haddon matrixes addressing the largely overlapping phenomena of violent youth gangs and violent political extremists (Tables II-3 and II-4). There appear to be important shared characteristics of these superficially different social problems. Both involve in-groups of persons who share an identity that is in conflict with one or more out-groups. Another similarity is that individuals who elect to participate are, in essence, electing a live-fast-die-young life history strategy (Victoroff et al., 2011). Another may be that both gang members and extremists are preoccupied with collective blame of others. It seems plausible that both urban youth and extremists may be propelled, to some degree, by audiovisual media depictions or incitement of violence (Tsfati, 2002; Atran and Stern, 2005; Gunter, 2008; Wright, 2008; Anderson et al., 2010). Moreover, it was recently reported that, just as elevated testosterone (T) levels are associated with antisocial behavior among adolescent boys, evidence suggests that elevated T may be associated with support for extremist violence among adolescent boys (Victoroff et al., 2011).

While it is tempting to propose a distinction—that youth gangs are not ideologically driven while extremist groups are—this overstates the difference. Although urban youth gangs may not base their violent plans on a coherent, articulated religious or political ideology, they clearly base their behaviors, in part, on a shared *weltanschauung* in which the local world is viewed as a hostile, hopeless, and insecure place in which conventional values are irrelevant, injustice is rampant, social Darwinism determines success, and in-group age-related gang affiliation offers identity, fictive kinship, and physical protection. Thus, gangsters evading the police in a crack house in Detroit or extremists evading drones in the souks of North Waziristan perhaps share the worldview of a beleaguered oppositional counterculture.

This is not by any means to say that urban youth gangs and violent extremist groups are identically structured or motivated. In conversations with members of Los Angeles gangs and with members of Hamas, both similarities and differences emerge. One important difference between these types of groups is that gang violence is often reactive—an immediate response to a confrontation with a rival, often unplanned, while terrorist

TABLE II-3 Haddon Matrix for Violent Urban Youth Gang Membership: Known or Suspected Risk Factors for the Occurrence and Dissemination of Gang-Related Violence

	Personal Factors	Vector or Agent Factors	Physical Environmental Factors	Social Environmental Factors	Policy Factors
Pre-event	• Gene variations impacting impulsivity, aggression, antisociality • Acquired differences in impulsivity, aggression, antisociality • Personal psychodynamics • Mood disorder • Proaggressive endophenotype • History of traumatic brain injury • ADHD • Autism spectrum disorder • Atypical steroid or peptide hormone metabolism • Other neuroatypicality • Perception of major loss • History of victimization • Frustration of aspirations	• Fetal environment • Environmental factors causing epigenetic variation • Childhood biological influences (e.g., lead exposure, malnutrition) • History of actual major loss • History of actual victimization • Media dissemination of violence and violent role models	• Dilapidated neighborhoods • Insufficient police presence • High ambient temperature and humidity • High housing density • Access to a motor vehicle • Anonymity afforded by large streets/freeways • Access to a weapon • Awareness of ready escape routes and hideouts	• Insufficient parental supervision • No successful noncriminal male role model • Childhood (especially familial) negative psychodynamic influences • Negative older sibling or peer influence • Social network influences • Widespread social disaffection • Social learning of violence • Lower socioeconomic status • Relative deprivation • Income inequity • Poor job prospects • Poor marriage prospects	• Inadequate funding for prenatal care • Inadequate funding for preschool education • Inadequate funding for day care • Inadequate funding for schools • Insufficient focus of schools on preparation for next-generation jobs • Inadequate funding for after-school programs • Inadequate funding for violence intervention programs • Inadequate funding for violence intervention research • National and local fiscal policy facilitating unemployment • Welfare and tax policies facilitating single motherhood • Right wing facilitation of nearly universal access to guns

TABLE II-3 Continued

Personal Factors	Vector or Agent Factors	Physical Environmental Factors	Social Environmental Factors	Policy Factors
• Attribution of that frustration to others • Need for identity consolidation • Perceived prejudice • Perceived injustice • Strong personal gang identity • Perceived need to defend gang status (e.g., to earn reputation or to escape from *leva*[a]) • Perceived financial need • Alienation from alternative identity groups (family, church, school, team) • Emotional state in the minutes prior to a confrontation			• Weak culture of scholastic achievement • Historical reasons for distrust of police and other authorities • Social prejudice • Social ignorance regarding the supposed deterrent efficacy of harsh sentencing • Reasons for the perpetrator to doubt the justice system • Strong gang in-group identity • Perception of gang and/or neighborhood collective jeopardy • Availability of a scapegoat	• Government facilitation of corporate arms sales • Lax oversight of media representations of violence • Inadequate oversight and correction of police and jail brutality • Political climate of disparaging minorities • Dysfunctional immigration policies • Political pressure for creating the appearance of being tough on crime • Mismatch between justice and sentencing guidelines • State emphasis on incarceration over rehabilitation • Vested political interests of law enforcement and prison guards • Political corruption supporting a movement to for-profit prisons

continued

TABLE II-3 Continued

	Personal Factors	Vector or Agent Factors	Physical Environmental Factors	Social Environmental Factors	Policy Factors
Event	• Neuroendocrine status at the time of confrontation • Autonomic nervous system status • Perceived threat • Attribution of ill intent • Perceived disrespect • Risk/benefit calculation • Perceived fiscal opportunity (e.g., shoes, jewelry, cars)	• Perceived vulnerability of targets	• Darkness • Isolation • Lack of video surveillance • Presence of attractive material goods	• Unplanned or planned encounter with out-group members • Special animus toward particular out-group members • Presence of peer gang witnesses • Presence of a female the actor wishes to impress • Absence of other witnesses	• Politically influenced maldistribution of law enforcement resources nearby the scene
Post-event	• Enhanced self-esteem or perceived glory • Relief of internal tension • Enhanced personal fiscal status (e.g., due to robbery) • Containment or denial of remorse	• Reinforcement of a narrative of the necessity of violent actions and the low risk of consequences	• Ready escape routes and hideouts • Limits on technology of tracking	• Enhanced in-group respect • Social promotion • Enhanced access to fertile females • Social networks supporting concealment	• Rarity of meaningful changes in gang-promoting public policies, even after the worst instances of gang violence

[a] *Leva* refers to being given the silent treatment by other gang members due to period infractions of the code of conduct.

TABLE II-4 Haddon Matrix for Violent Extremist Groups: Known or Suspected Risk Factors for the Occurrence and Dissemination of Political Violence

	Personal Factors	Vector or Agent Factors	Physical Environmental Factors	Social Environmental Factors	Policy Factors
Pre-event	• Gene variations impacting in-group affiliation/out-group derogation, perceived injustice, moral certainty, aggression • Acquired variations in in-group affiliation/out-group derogation, perceived injustice, moral certainty, aggression • Pro-aggressive endophenotype • Personal psychodynamics • Depression • Frustration of aspirations • Attribution of that frustration to political out-group • Atypical steroid or peptide hormone metabolism	• Fetal environment • Environmental factors causing epigenetic variation • Childhood biological influences • History of actual major life losses • History of actual victimization by out-group • Media dissemination/ glorification of extremist ideology and actions	• Inadequate physical defenses • Insufficient police/ military presence • Ability to travel • Anonymity afforded by large cities • Access to weapons, including WMDs • Awareness of ready escape routes and hideouts	• Childhood (especially familial) psychodynamic influences • Widespread social disaffection • Social learning of violence • Positive social image of extremist role models • Communal support for extremist group • Social network influences • Exposure to charismatic ideologues • Collective moral condemnation of out-group • Fear of challenges to social or sexual order from out-group • Perceived social injustice	• Political oppression • Systematic prejudice in laws, housing, education, or employment against out-groups • Educational systems biased against out-groups • Government facilitation of corporate arms sales • Mismatch between a government's stated and actual values • Poor control of media representations of terrorist ideology and behavior • Out-group police, military, and judicial policies blind to justice or likely to be interpreted as unjust

continued

TABLE II-4 Continued

	Personal Factors	Vector or Agent Factors	Physical Environmental Factors	Social Environmental Factors	Policy Factors
Pre-event	• Neuroatypicality • Perception of major loss • Perception of victimization • Need for identity consolidation • Perceived prejudice • Perceived injustice • Perceived need to prove oneself to group • Strong personal extremist in-group identity • Frequent religious observance			• Perceived threat against the in-group • Perceived social or religious requirement for extremist behaviors • Historical reasons to distrust authorities • Actual social prejudice • Poor job prospects • Poor marriage prospects • Strong culture of antisocial punishment • Historical disputes over territory/resources • Inadequate defensive intelligence • Strong extremist in-group identity • Groupthink denying risk and vulnerabilities	• Poor oversight and correction of police and jail brutality • Political climate of disparaging minorities • Failure of moderation of political rhetoric about the in-group by the out-group[a] • Dysfunctional immigration policies • Discriminatory laws • Unilateral actions by the out-group, especially those likely to be perceived as arrogant, culturally insensitive, or unjust • Institutional failures to recognize connections between government policies and extremism

TABLE II-4 Continued

	Personal Factors	Vector or Agent Factors	Physical Environmental Factors	Social Environmental Factors	Policy Factors
Pre-event				• Out-group cultural insensitivity • Out-group resistance to examining the justice of their own actions	• Occupation of or other violations of sovereignty (e.g., political meddling, targeted assassinations, presence of military "advisors," drone attacks, etc.) • Imposition of alien political systems such as "democracy"
Event	• Neuroendocrine status at the time of attacks • Autonomic nervous system status • Emotional status • Sufficient self control for risky or suicidal militant action	• Perceived vulnerability of targets	• Physical access to target	• Usually carefully planned encounter with out-group representatives; presence of peer witnesses; sluggish, poorly coordinated defensive responses	• Politically influenced gaps in defense

continued

TABLE II-4 Continued

	Personal Factors	Vector or Agent Factors	Physical Environmental Factors	Social Environmental Factors	Policy Factors
Post-event	• Enhanced self-esteem and/or perceived glory • Satisfaction • Relief of internal tension • Containment or denial of remorse		• Ready escape routes and hideouts • Foreign safe havens • Limits on technology of tracking	• Enhanced in-group respect • Social promotion • Enhanced access to fertile females • Social networks supporting concealment	• Ineffectual focus on retaliation • Pandering to domestic political agendas at the expense of evaluating and addressing root causes and impartial empirical analysis of effectiveness of current strategies

[a] E.g., Bush, 2001, "this *crusade*, this war on terrorism is going to take a while."

aggression is more likely to be proactive and premeditated. Even so, just as extremists usually plan their attacks, gangs sometime premeditate attacks or lie in wait. Another difference is that urban street gangs usually comprise age-stratified networks, while extremist networks are less likely to be age stratified. Another difference is that, while members of urban gangs would die to defend their fictive brothers, they are not devoted to advancing an ideological goal that would benefit a significant part of society as much as they are devoted to advancing their own personal interests, including entrepreneurial ambitions. That is, while young people ultimately join any type of violent group out of personal interest, that interest is conscious and explicit in the case of urban gangsters, but not among violent extremists. Another possible difference relates to perceived progress toward life goals, hope, and well-being; while frustration is expressed by both gang members and extremists, acknowledging a lack of quantitative empirical evidence, it is my impression that there is more fatalism and anomie among typical urban gang members and more hope (realistic or not) of a changed world among extremists. This is perhaps consistent with the empirical observation of relatively high rates of depression and anxiety among members of youth gangs—a phenomenon that perhaps relates, in part, to another difference: youth gang members are at a high rate of victimization in their communities (Taylor et al., 2008).

In these preliminary Haddon matrixes, the content of each cell is based on empirical research, but does not provide weightings in terms of scientific defensibility for each proposed causal factor. Instead, these are known or suspected causal factors for which the literature supports further investigation (for the sake of concision in this brief essay, I will not offer citations for each factor in each cell; such citations are available on request).

It is immediately apparent that known or suspected causal factors might sometimes be assigned to more than one cell. For example, heritable environmentally induced epigenetic changes favoring impulsivity, aggression, hyperresponsiveness or threat, irritability, group allegiance, or urge for antisocial punishment could be classified as *Vectors* or *Agents* that disseminate violent gang behavior, but, once present in somatic cells, might also be classified as *Individual* factors. One must rush to acknowledge the relative paucity of empirical findings supporting the influence of the proposed factors in Tables II-3 and II-4. The biggest challenge is to identify the vector. That is, if violent behaviors, like injuries, occur in contagious clusters, it would be valuable to identify the mechanism of transmission.

Conclusion

In conclusion, natural selection is responsible for the human population as it is. Human brains mediate both individual and collective violent behaviors because those behaviors proved active in the ancestral environment. Self-recruitment to aggressive groups—whether Seal Team 6, al Qaeda, or the Crips—occurs largely for the same reasons: late adolescents and young adults, men more than women, have brains that arrive at the largely unconscious conclusion that being seen to participate in violence against an out-group makes one worthy of the rewards of reciprocal altruism. Violence and altruism are not polar opposites, but two sides of the same coin of evolved, adaptive human nature.

It is self-evident that innate and acquired biological factors interact with environmental factors to determine who will become a violent criminal, a gangster, or a terrorist. That indisputable observation does not relieve us of the responsibility to determine how this occurs, and what elements of the causal algorithm are susceptible to what cost-effective interventions. Political agendas probably represent a barrier to the mitigation of violence. Yet rigorous empirical research holds the promise of informing better violence prevention policies. This will be the work of generations.

REFERENCES

Adams, D. B. 2006. Brain mechanisms of aggressive behavior: An updated review. *Neuroscience and Biobehavioral Reviews* 30(3):304-318.

Adler, J. S. 2003. "We've got a right to fight; we're married": Domestic homicide in Chicago, 1875-1920. *Journal of Interdisciplinary History* 34(1):27-48.

Amnesty International. 1997. *Amnesty International report 1997.* London, UK: Amnesty International, International Secretariat.

Amnesty International. 2004. *Lives blown apart: Crimes against women in times of conflict, stop violence against women.* London, UK: Amnesty International, International Secretariat.

Amnesty International. 2008. *Amnesty International report 2008: The state of the world's human rights.* New York: Amnesty International USA.

Anderson, C. A., A. Shibuya, N. Ihori, E. L. Swing, B. J. Bushman, A. Sakamoto, H. R. Rothstein, and M. Saleem. 2010. Violent video game effects on aggression, empathy, and prosocial behavior in eastern and western countries: A meta-analytic review. *Psychological Bulletin* 136(2):151-173.

Anderson, R. M., and R. M. May. 1991. *Infectious diseases of humans: Dynamics and control.* New York: Oxford University Press.

Annan, J., C. Blattman, and R. Horton. 2006. *The state of youth and youth protection in Northern Uganda: Findings from the survey of war affected youth.* Kampala, Uganda: UNICEF.

Archer, D., and R. Gartner. 1976. Violent acts and violent times: A comparative approach to postwar homicide rates. *American Sociology Review* 41(6):937-963.

Archer, D., and R. Gartner. 1984. *Violence and crime in cross-national perspective.* New Haven, CT: Yale University Press.

Atran, S., and J. Stern. 2005. Small groups find fatal purpose through the Web. *Nature* 437(7059):620.

Avenanti, A., D. Bueti, G. Galati, and S. M. Aglioti. 2005. Transcranial magnetic stimulation highlights the sensorimotor side of empathy for pain. *Nature Neuroscience* 8(7):955-960.

Aziz-Zadeh, L., F. Maeda, E. Zaidel, J. Mazziotta, and M. Iacoboni. 2002. Lateralization in motor facilitation during action observation: A TMS study. *Experimental Brain Research* 144(1):127-131.

Baker, F. M., and C. C. Bell. 1999. African Americans: Treatment concerns. *Psychiatric Services* 50:362-368.

Bandura, A. 1973. Social learning theory of aggression. In *The control of aggression: Implications from basic research*, edited by J. F. Knutson. Hawthorne, NY: Aldine.

Bandura, A. 1977. *Social learning theory.* Englewood Cliffs, NJ: Prentice Hall.

Bandura, A. 1986. *Social foundations of thought and action: A social cognitive theory.* Englewood Cliffs, NJ: Prentice Hall.

Bandura, A., and A. C. Huston. 1961. Identification as a process of incidental learning. *Journal of Abnormal and Social Psychology* 63(2):311-318.

Bandura, A., S. A. Ross, and D. Ross. 1961. Transmission of aggression through imitation of aggressive models. *Journal of Abnormal and Social Psychology* 63(3):575-582.

Barber, B. K., ed. 2009. *Adolescents and war: How youth deal with political violence.* New York: Oxford University Press.

Barclay, P., and R. Willer. 2007. Partner choice creates competitive altruism in humans. *Proceedings of the Royal Society B-Biological Sciences* 274(1610):749-753.

Barkin, S., S. Kreiter, and R. H. DuRant. 2001. Exposure to violence and intentions to engage in moralistic violence during early adolescence. *Journal of Adolescence* 24(6):777-789.

Baumeister, R. F., and M. R. Leary. 1995. The need to belong: Desire for interpersonal attachments as a fundamental human-motivation. *Psychological Bulletin* 117(3):497-529.

Bell, C. C. 1986. Coma and the etiology of violence, part 1. *Journal of the National Medical Association* 78(12):1167-1176.

Bell, C. C. 1987. Coma and the etiology of violence, part 2. *Journal of the National Medical Association* 79(1):79-85.

Bell, C. C. 1997. Community violence: Causes, prevention, and intervention. *Journal of the National Medical Association* 89(10):657-662.

Bell, C. C. 2001. Cultivating resiliency in youth. *Journal of Adolescent Health* 29(5):375-381.

Bell, C. C. 2012. Preventing fetal alcohol syndrome. *Clinical Psychiatry News* 40(5).

Bell, C. C., and R. P. Kelly. 1987. Head injury with subsequent, intermittent, nonschizophrenic, psychotic symptoms and violence. *Journal of the National Medical Association* 79(11):1139-1144.

Bell, C. C., and D. F. McBride. 2010a. Commentary on Bourget D, Gagné, Whitehurst L. Domestic homicide and homicide-suicide: The older offender. *Journal of the American Academy of Psychiatry and the Law* 38(3):312-317.

Bell, C. C., and D. F. McBride. 2010b. Affect regulation and the prevention of risky behaviors. *Journal of the American Medical Association* 304(5):565-566.

Bell, C. C., B. Thompson, K. Shorter-Gooden, B. Shakoor, D. Dew, E. Hughley, and R. Mays. 1985. Prevalence of episodes of coma in black subjects. *Journal of the National Medical Association* 77(5):391-395.

Bell, C. C., A. Bhana, I. Petersen, M. M. McKay, R. Gibbons, W. Bannon, and A. Amatya. 2008. Building protective factors to offset sexually risky behaviors among black youths: A randomized control trial. *Journal of the National Medical Association* 100(8):936-944.

Berman, S. L., W. M. Kurtines, W. K. Silverman, and L. T. Serafini. 1996. The impact of exposure to crime and violence on urban youth. *American Journal of Orthopsychiatry* 66(3):329-336.

Berry, J. W. 2001. A psychology of immigration. *Journal of Social Issues* 57(3):615-631.

132

CONTAGION OF VIOLENCE

Betancourt, T. S., R. T. Brennan, J. Rubin-Smith, G. M. Fitzmaurice, and S. E. Gilman. 2010. Sierra Leone's former child soldiers: A longitudinal study of risk, protective factors, and mental health. *Journal of the American Academy of Child and Adolescent Psychiatry* 49(6):606-615.

Bien, N., A. Roebroeck, R. Goebel, and A. T. Sack. 2009. The brain's intention to imitate: The neurobiology of intentional versus automatic imitation. *Cerebral Cortex* 19(10): 2338-2351.

BJS (Bureau of Justice Statistics). 2005. *Homicide trends in the United States; long term trends.* http://bjs.ojp.usdoj.gov/content/homicide/tables/totalstab.cfm (accessed on September 13, 2012).

BJS. 2011. *U.S. correctional population declined for second consecutive year.* Washington, DC: Bureau of Justice Statistics.

Bohstedt, J. 1994. The dynamics of riots: Escalation and diffusion/contagion. In *The dynamics of aggression: Biological and social processes in dyads and groups,* edited by J. Bohstedt. Hillsdale, NJ: Lawrence Erlbaum Associates.

Bowles, S. 2009. Did warfare among ancestral hunter-gatherers affect the evolution of human social behaviors? *Science* 324(5932):1293-1298.

Boxer, P., L. Rowell Huesmann, E. F. Dubow, S. F. Landau, S. D. Gvirsman, K. Shikaki, and J. Ginges. 2012. Exposure to violence across the social ecosystem and the development of aggression: A test of ecological theory in the Israeli-Palestinian conflict. *Child Development* [Epub ahead of print].

Boxford, S. 2006. Schools and the problem of crime. Devon, UK: Willan Publishing.

Brass, M., J. Derrfuss, and D. Y. von Cramon. 2005. The inhibition of imitative and over-learned responses: A functional double dissociation. *Neuropsychologia* 43(1):89-98.

Brent, D. A., M. M. Kerr, C. Goldstein, J. Bozigar, M. Wartella, and M. J. Allan. 1989. An outbreak of suicide and suicidal-behavior in a high-school. *Journal of the American Academy of Child and Adolescent Psychiatry* 28(6):918-924.

Bronfenbrenner, U. 1979. *The ecology of human development: Experiments by nature and design.* Cambridge, MA: The Harvard University Press.

Bronfenbrenner, U. 2005. Making human beings human: Bioecological perspectives on human development. In *The Sage program on applied developmental science.* Thousand Oaks, CA: Sage Publications.

Bruneau, E. G., N. Dufour, and R. Saxe. 2012. Social cognition in members of conflict groups: Behavioural and neural responses in Arabs, Israelis and South Americans to each other's misfortunes. *Philosophical Transactions of the Royal Society B-Biological Sciences* 367(1589):717-730.

Bukstel, L. H., and P. R. Kilmann. 1980. Psychological Effects of Imprisonment on Confined Individuals. *Psychological Bulletin* 88(2):469-493.

Campbell, G. R. 2010. *Many Americas: Critical perspectives on race, racism, and ethnicity.* Dubuque, IA: Kendall/Hunt Publishing Company.

Carr, L., M. Iacoboni, M. C. Dubeau, J. C. Mazziotta, and G. L. Lenzi. 2003. Neural mechanisms of empathy in humans: A relay from neural systems for imitation to limbic areas. *PNAS* 100(9):5497-5502.

Catani, C., E. Schauer, and F. Neuner. 2008. Beyond individual war trauma: Domestic violence against children in Afghanistan and Sri Lanka. *Journal of Marital and Family Therapy* 34(2):165-176.

Catani, C., E. Schauer, T. Elbert, I. Missmahl, J. P. Bette, and F. Neuner. 2009. War trauma, child labor, and family violence: Life adversities and PTSD in a sample of school children in Kabul. *Journal of Traumatic Stress* 22(3):163-171.

Cavanaugh, C. E., J. T. Messing, M. Del-Colle, C. O'Sullivan, and J. C. Campbell. 2011. Prevalence and correlates of suicidal behavior among adult female victims of intimate partner violence. *Suicide and Life Threatening Behavior* 41(4):372-383.

Champagne, D. 2012. Justice and consensus. *Indian Country* 2(19):16.

Chen, Y. Y., P. C. Tsai, P. H. Chen, C. C. Fan, G. Hung, and A. T. A. Cheng. 2010. Effect of media reporting of the suicide of a singer in Taiwan: The case of Ivy Li. *Social Psychiatry and Psychiatric Epidemiology* 45(3):363-369.

Chen, Y. Y., S. F. Liao, P. R. Teng, C. W. Tsai, H. F. Fan, W. C. Lee, and A. T. A. Cheng. 2012. The impact of media reporting of the suicide of a singer on suicide rates in Taiwan. *Social Psychiatry and Psychiatric Epidemiology* 47(2):215-221.

Cheng, A. T. A., K. Hawton, T. H. H. Chen, A. M. F. Yen, J. C. Chang, M. Y. Chong, C. Y. Liu, Y. Lee, P. R. Teng, and L. C. Chen. 2007a. The influence of media reporting of a celebrity suicide on suicidal behavior in patients with a history of depressive disorder. *Journal of Affective Disorders* 103(1-3):69-75.

Cheng, A. T. A., K. Hawton, C. T. C. Lee, and T. H. H. Chen. 2007b. The influence of media reporting of the suicide of a celebrity on suicide rates: A population-based study. *International Journal of Epidemiology* 36(6):1229-1234.

Cheng, Q. J., F. Chen, and P. S. F. Yip. 2011. The Foxconn suicides and their media prominence: Is the Werther effect applicable in China? *BMC Public Health* 11:841.

Chung, R. C.-Y. 2001. Psychosocial adjustment of Cambodian refugee women: Implications for mental health counseling. *Journal of Mental Health Counseling* 23(2):115.

CIET Africa. 2004. *Sexual violence and HIV/AIDS. Executive report on the 2002 nationwide youth survey.*

Cisek, P., and J. F. Kalaska. 2004. Neural correlates of mental rehearsal in dorsal premotor cortex. *Nature* 431(7011):993-996.

City of Chicago. *City of Chicago data portal.* https://data.cityofchicago.org (accessed October 1, 2012).

Clark, C. J., S. A. Everson-Rose, S. F. Suglia, R. Btoush, A. Alonso, and M. M. Haj-Yahia. 2010. Association between exposure to political violence and intimate-partner violence in the occupied Palestinian territory: A cross-sectional study. *Lancet* 375(9711):310-316.

Cohen, D. 2010. Probabilistic epigenesis: An alternative causal model for conduct disorders in children and adolescents. *Neuroscience and Biobehavioral Reviews* 34(1):119-129.

Coid, J., A. Petruckevitch, G. Feder, W. S. Chung, J. Richardson, and S. Moorey. 2001. Relation between childhood sexual and physical abuse and risk of revictimisation in women: A cross-sectional survey. *Lancet* 358(9280):450-454.

Cole, E., E. D. Rothblum, and O. M. Espin, eds. 1993. *Refugee women and their mental health: Shattered societies, shattered lives.* Binghampton, NY: Haworth Press, Inc.

Comai, S., M. Tau, and G. Gobbi. 2012. The psychopharmacology of aggressive behavior: A translational approach part 1: Neurobiology. *Journal of Clinical Psychopharmacology* 32(1):83-94.

Cox, D. 1987. The migration-integration process. In *Migration and welfare: An Australian perspective.* Sydney, Australia: Prentice Hall.

Crenshaw, M. 1986. The psychology of political terrorism. In *Political psychology*, edited by M. Hermann. San Francisco, CA: Jossey-Bass Publishers.

Crenshaw, M. 1995. Thoughts on relating terrorism to historical contexts. In *Terrorism in context*, edited by M. Crenshaw. University Park, PA: The Pennsylvania State University Press.

Crenshaw, M. 2000. The psychology of terrorism: An agenda for the 21st century. *Political Psychology* 21(2):405-420.

Crooks, C. V., K. L. Scott, D. A. Wolfe, D. Chiodo, and S. Killip. 2007. Understanding the link between childhood maltreatment and violent delinquency: What do schools have to add? *Child Maltreatment* 12(3):269-280.

Cross, K. A., and M. Iacoboni. 2011. Optimized neural coding? Control mechanisms in large cortical networks implemented by connectivity changes. *Human Brain Mapping* [Epub ahead of print].

Cummings, E. M., A. C. Schermerhorn, C. E. Merrilees, M. C. Goeke-Morey, P. Shirlow, and E. Cairns. 2010. Political violence and child adjustment in Northern Ireland: Testing pathways in a social-ecological model including single- and two-parent families. *Developmental Psychology* 46(4):827-841.

Cummings, E. M., C. E. Merrilees, A. C. Schermerhorn, M. C. Goeke-Morey, P. Shirlow, and E. Cairns. 2011. Longitudinal pathways between political violence and child adjustment: The role of emotional security about the community in Northern Ireland. *Journal of Abnormal Child Psychology* 39(2):213-224.

Cutler, D. M., E. L. Glaesen, and K. E. Norberg. 2001. Explaining the rise in youth suicide. In *Risky behavior among youths: An economic analysis*, edited by J. Gruber. Chicago, IL: University of Chicago Press.

Dapretto, M., M. S. Davies, J. H. Pfeifer, A. A. Scott, M. Sigman, S. Y. Bookheimer, and M. Iacoboni. 2006. Understanding emotions in others: Mirror neuron dysfunction in children with autism spectrum disorders. *Nature Neuroscience* 9(1):28-30.

Davidson, L. E., M. L. Rosenberg, J. A. Mercy, J. Franklin, and J. T. Simmons. 1989. An epidemiologic study of risk factors in two teenage suicide clusters. *JAMA* 262(19):2687-2692.

De Jong, J. 2010. A public health framework to translate risk factors related to political violence and war into multi-level preventive interventions. *Social Science & Medicine* 70(1):71-79.

De Kruif, P. 1926. *Microbe hunters*. New York: Harcourt, Brace and Co.

De Renzi, E., F. Cavalleri, and S. Facchini. 1996. Imitation and utilisation behaviour. *Journal of Neurology, Neurosurgery and Psychiatry* 61(4):396-400.

Debarbiaux, E. 2003. School violence in Europe: Discussion, knowledge and uncertainty. In *Council of Europe violence in schools: A challenge for the local community*. Luxembourg: Council of Europe Publications.

Decker, S. H. 1996. Collective and normative features of gang violence. *Justice Quarterly* 13(2):243-264.

Devries, K., C. Watts, M. Yoshihama, L. Kiss, L. B. Schraiber, N. Deyessa, L. Heise, J. Durand, J. Mbwambo, H. Jansen, Y. Berhane, M. Ellsberg, and C. Garcia-Moreno. 2011. Violence against women is strongly associated with suicide attempts: Evidence from the WHO multi-country study on women's health and domestic violence against women. *Social Science and Medicine* 73(1):79-86.

Dipellegrino, G., L. Fadiga, L. Fogassi, V. Gallese, and G. Rizzolatti. 1992. Understanding motor events: A neurophysiological study. *Experimental Brain Research* 91(1):176-180.

DOJ (U.S. Department of Justice). 2009. CeaseFire: A public health approach to reduce shootings and killings. *NIJ Journal* 264.

DOJ. 2011. *National Crime Victimization Survey: Criminal victimization, 2010*, http://bjs.ojp.usdoj.gov/index.cfm?ty=dcdetail&iid=245 (accessed August 20, 2012).

Dorland, W. A. N. 2010. *Dorland's illustrated medical dictionary*. 32nd ed. Philadelphia, PA: Saunders/Elsevier.

Dossa, P. 2004. *Politics and the poetics of migration: Narratives of Iranian women from the diaspora*. Toronto, Canada: Canadian Scholars' Press.

Dossa, P. 2010. Exploring the disjuncture between the politics of trauma and everyday realities of women in Afghanistan. *Journal of Muslim Mental Health* 5(1):8-21.

Douglas, K., and C. C. Bell. 2011. Violence prevention in youth. *Psychiatric Clinics of North America—Prevention in Psychiatry* 34(3):205-216.

Dowling, H. F. 1977. *Fighting infection: Conquests of the twentieth century.* Cambridge, MA: Harvard University Press.

Dubow, E. F., L. R. Huesmann, and P. Boxer. 2009. A social-cognitive-ecological framework for understanding the impact of exposure to persistent ethnic-political violence on children's psychosocial adjustment. *Clinical Child and Family Psychology Review* 12(2):113-126.

Dubow, E. F., P. Boxer, L. R. Huesmann, K. Shikaki, S. Landau, S. D. Gvirsman, and J. Ginges. 2010. Exposure to conflict and violence across contexts: Relations to adjustment among Palestinian children. *Journal of Clinical Child and Adolescent Psychology* 39(1):103-116.

Dubow, E. F., P. Boxer, L. R. Huesmann, S. F. Landau, S. D. Gvirsman, K. Shikaki, and J. Ginges. 2011. *Mediators of the relation between exposure to violence and aggression in Israeli and Palestinian youths.* Presented at the 2011 Biennial Meeting of the Society for Research in Child Development, Montreal, April 2, 2011.

DuRant, R. H., R. A. Pendergrast, and C. Cadenhead. 1994. Exposure to violence and victimization and fighting behavior by urban black-adolescents *Journal of Adolescent Health* 15(4):311-318.

DuRant, R. H., F. Treiber, E. Goodman, and E. R. Woods. 1996. Intentions to use violence among young adolescents. *Pediatrics* 98(6):1104-1108.

Dushanova, J., and J. Donoghue. 2010. Neurons in primary motor cortex engaged during action observation. *European Journal of Neuroscience* 31(2):386-398.

Economist. 2008. *The world in 2009.* Westminster, UK: The Economist Group.

Economist Intelligence Unit. 2009. The political instability index: Social unrest. *Economist.* http://viewswire.eiu.com/site_info.asp?info_name=social_unrest_table&page=noads (accessed August 1, 2012).

Ehrensaft, M. K., P. Cohen, J. Brown, E. Smailes, H. N. Chen, and J. G. Johnson. 2003. Intergenerational transmission of partner violence: A 20-year prospective study. *Journal of Consulting and Clinical Psychology* 71(4):741-753.

Eisenberger, N. I. 2011. Why rejection hurts: What social neuroscience has revealed about the brain's response to social rejection. In *The handbook of social neuroscience,* edited by C. J. Decety. New York: Oxford University Press.

Eisenberger, N. I. 2012. The neural bases of social pain: Evidence for shared representations with physical pain. *Psychosomatic Medicine* 74(2):126-135.

Eisenberger, N. I., and M. D. Lieberman. 2004. Why rejection hurts: A common neural alarm system for physical and social pain. *Trends in Cognitive Science* 8(7):294-300.

Eisenberger, N. I., and M. D. Lieberman. 2005. Broken hearts and broken bones: The neurocognitive overlap between social pain and physical pain. In *The social outcast: Ostracism, social exclusion, rejection, and bullying,* edited by K. D. Williams, J. P. Forgas, and W. von Hippel. New York: Cambridge University Press.

Ellis, D., H. G. Grasmick, and B. Gilman. 1974. Violence in prisons: A sociological analysis. *American Journal of Sociology* 80(1):16-43.

Etzersdorfer, E., G. Sonneck, and S. Nagelkuess. 1992. Newspaper reports and suicide. *New England Journal of Medicine* 327(7):502-503.

Etzersdorfer, E., M. Voracek, and G. Sonneck. 2004. A dose-response relationship between imitational suicides and newspaper distribution. *Archives of Suicide Research* 8(2):137-145.

Fadiga, L., L. Fogassi, G. Pavesi, and G. Rizzolatti. 1995. Motor facilitation during action observation: magnetic stimulation study. *Journal of Neurophysiology* 73(6):2608-2611.

Fagan, J., and G. Davies. 2004. The natural history of neighborhood violence. *Journal of Contemporary Criminal Justice* 20(2):127-147.

Fagan, J., F. E. Zimring, and J. Kim. 1998. Declining homicide in New York City: A tale of two trends. *Journal of Criminal Law & Criminology* 88(4):1277-1323.

Fagan, J., D. L. Wilkinson, and G. Davies. 2007. Social contagion of violence. In *The Cambridge handbook of violent behavior*, edited by D. Flannery.

Farah, A. H., K. H. Aaden, C. Bentley, S. Gove, A. Ali-Salaad, and G. Slutkin. 1985. *The Cholera epidemic in the Northwest Regions of Somalia, March-April, 1985*. Official Report of the Cholera control Committee (Hargeisa). Somali Democratic Republic.

FBI (Federal Bureau of Investigation). 2008. *Uniform crime reports*. http://www.fbi.gov/about-us/cjis/ucr/ucr (accessed September 13, 2012).

Fekete, S., A. Schmidtke, Y. Takahashi, E. Etzersdorfer, M. Upanne, and P. Osvath. 2001. Mass media, cultural attitudes, and suicide. Results of an international comparative study. *Crisis: The Journal of Crisis Intervention and Suicide Prevention* 22(4):170-172.

Finch, B. K., B. Kolody, and W. A. Vega. 2000. Perceived discrimination and depression among Mexican-origin adults in California. *Journal of Health and Social Behavior* 41(3):295-313.

Fogassi, L., P. F. Ferrari, B. Gesierich, S. Rozzi, F. Chersi, and G. Rizzolatti. 2005. Parietal lobe: From action organization to intention understanding. *Science* 308(5722):662-667.

Fonzo, G. A., A. N. Simmons, S. R. Thorp, S. B. Norman, M. P. Paulus, and M. B. Stein. 2010. Exaggerated and disconnected insular-amygdalar blood oxygenation level-dependent response to threat-related emotional faces in women with intimate-partner violence posttraumatic stress disorder. *Biological Psychiatry* 68(5):433-441.

Fox, J. 2004. Is ethnoreligious conflict a contagious disease? *Studies in Conflict and Terrorism* 27(2):89-106.

Fries, A. B. W., T. E. Ziegler, J. R. Kurian, S. Jacoris, and S. D. Pollak. 2005. Early experience in humans is associated with changes in neuropeptides critical for regulating social behavior. *Proceedings of the National Academy of Sciences USA* 102(47):17237-17240.

Gallese, V., L. Fadiga, L. Fogassi, and G. Rizzolatti. 1996. Action recognition in the premotor cortex. *Brain* 119:593-609.

Garbino, J., C. P. Bradshaw, and J. A. Vorrasi. 2002. Mitigating the effects of gun violence on children and youth. *The Future of Children* 12:73-85.

Garrod, S., and M. J. Pickering. 2004. Why is conversation so easy? *Trends in Cognitive Science* 8(1):8-11.

Gentilucci, M., L. Fogassi, G. Luppino, M. Matelli, R. Camarda, and G. Rizzolatti. 1988. Functional-organization of inferior area-6 in the macaque monkey. Somatotopy and the control of proximal movements. *Experimental Brain Research* 71(3):475-490.

Gilligan, J. 1997. *Violence: Reflections on a national epidemic*, edited by 1st Vintage Books. New York: Vintage Books.

Gottfredson, D. C. 2001. *Schools and delinquency*. Cambridge, UK: Cambridge University Press.

Gould, M. S. 1990. Suicide clusters and media exposure. In *Suicide over the life cycle: Risk factors, assessment, and treatment of suicidal patients*, edited by S. Blumenthal and D. Kupfer. Washington, DC: American Psychiatric Association. Pp. 517-532.

Gould, M. S. 2001. Suicide and the media. In *Clinical science of suicide prevention*. Vol. 932, *Annals of the New York Academy of Sciences*, edited by H. Hendin and J. J. Mann. New York: New York Academy of Sciences.

Gould, M. S., S. Wallenstein, and L. Davidson. 1989. Suicide clusters: A critical-review. *Suicide and Life-Threatening Behavior* 19(1):17-29.

Gould, M. S., S. Wallenstein, M. H. Kleinman, P. Ocarroll, and J. Mercy. 1990. Suicide clusters: An examination of age-specific effects. *American Journal of Public Health* 80(2):211-212.

Gould, M. S., T. Greenberg, D. M. Velting, and D. Shaffer. 2003. Youth suicide risk and preventive interventions: A review of the past 10 years. *Journal of the American Academy of Child and Adolescent Psychiatry* 42(4):386-405.

Gould, M. S., F. A. Marrocco, K. Hoagwood, M. Kleinman, L. Amakawa, and E. Altschuler. 2009. Service use by at-risk youths after school-based suicide screening. *Journal of the American Academy of Child and Adolescent Psychiatry* 48(12):1193-1201.

Gozdiak, E. M. 2009. Culturally competent responses to the effects of armed conflict on well-being on refugee women. In *Women, migration and conflict: Breaking a deadly cycle*, edited by S. Forbes Marton and J. Tirman. New York: Springer.

Gozdiak, E. M., and K. C. Long. 2005. *Suffering and resiliency of refugee women: An annotated bibliography 1980-2005*. Institute for the Study of International Migration (ISIM), Georgetown University. http://isim.georgetown.edu/publications/2005_Suffering_and_Resiliency.pdf (accessed August 1, 2012).

Green, M., D. Thomas, W. Ball, and M. Gareth. 1982. *Koch centennial memorial: 100th anniversary, announcement of the discovery of the tubercle bacillus by Robert Koch, March 24, 1882*. New York: American Lung Association.

Greenfield, L. A., M. R. Rand, D. Craven, P. A. Klaus, C. A. Perkins, C. Ringel, G. Warchol, C. Maston, and J. A. Fox. 1998. *Violence by intimates*. Washington, DC: US Department of Justice, Office of Justice Programs, Bureau of Justice Statistics.

Griffin, G., E. McEwen, B. H. Samuels, H. Suggs, J. L. Redd, and G. M. McClelland. 2011. Infusing protective factors for children in foster care. *Psychiatric Clinics of North America* 34(1):185-203.

Guerra, N. G., L. R. Huesmann, and A. Spindler. 2003. Community violence exposure, social cognition, and aggression among urban elementary school children. *Child Development* 74(5):1561-1576.

Gunter, B. 2008. Media violence: Is there a case for causality? *American Behavioral Scientist* 51(8):1061-1122.

Hacker, K., J. Collins, L. Gross-Young, S. Almeida, and N. Burke. 2008. Coping with youth suicide and overdose—one community's efforts to investigate, intervene, and prevent suicide contagion. *Crisis: The Journal of Crisis Intervention and Suicide Prevention* 29(2):86-95.

Hagihara, A., K. Tarumi, and T. Abe. 2007. Media suicide-reports, Internet use and the occurrence of suicides between 1987 and 2005 in Japan. *BMC Public Health* 7.

Haney, C. 2002. *The psychological impact of incarceration: Implications for post-prison adjustment*. Paper presented at From Prisons to Home Conference, National Institutes of Health: Bethesda, MD. January 30-31.

Hanson, R. F., S. Self-Brown, A. Fricker-Elhai, D. G. Kilpatrick, B. E. Saunders, and H. Resnick. 2006. Relations among parental substance use, violence exposure and mental health: The national survey of adolescents. *Addiction Behavior* 31(11):1988-2001.

Hari, R., N. Forss, S. Avikainen, E. Kirveskari, S. Salenius, and G. Rizzolatti. 1998. Activation of human primary motor cortex during action observation: A neuromagnetic study. *Proceedings of the National Academy of Sciences USA* 95(25):15061-15065.

Hawton, K., S. Simkin, J. J. Deeks, S. O'Connor, A. Keen, D. G. Altman, G. Philo, and C. Bulstrode. 1999. Effects of a drug overdose in a television drama on presentations to hospital for self poisoning: Time series and questionnaire study. *BMJ* 318(7189):972-977.

Hawton, K., L. Harriss, and K. Rodham. 2010. How adolescents who cut themselves differ from those who take overdoses. *European Child & Adolescent Psychiatry* 19(6):513-523.

Hazell, P. 1993. Adolescent suicide clusters—evidence, mechanisms and prevention. *Australian and New Zealand Journal of Psychiatry* 27(4):653-665.

Health Care Innovations Exchange Team. 2012. *Preventing and mitigating the effects of childhood violence and trauma: An interview with Carl C. Bell, M.D.* http://www.innovations.ahrq.gov/content.aspx?id=3382 (accessed August 1, 2012).

Heyman, R. E., and A. M. S. Slep. 2002. Do child abuse and interparental violence lead to adulthood family violence? *Journal of Marriage and Family* 64(4):864-870.

Heymann, D. L. 2008. *Control of communicable diseases manual*, 19th ed. Edited by D. L. Heymann. Washington, DC: American Public Health Association.

HHS (U.S. Department of Health and Human Services). 2001. *Youth violence: a report of the Surgeon General.* Rockville, MD: Department of Health and Human Services.

HHS. 2010. *Suicide Prevention Research in Indian Country.* Office of Minority Health. http://minorityhealth.hhs.gov (accessed August 1, 2012).

HHS. 2011. American Indian/Alaska Native national behavioral health strategic plan, 2011-2015. http://www.ihs.gov (accessed August 1, 2012).

Hill, A. B. 1965. Environment and disease-association or causation. *Proceedings of the Royal Society of Medicine-London* 58(5):295-300.

Huesmann, L. R. 2010. Nailing the coffin shut on doubts that violent video games stimulate aggression: Comment on Anderson et al. (2010). *Psychological Bulletin* 136(2):179-181.

Huesmann, L. R., and L. D. Eron. 1984. Cognitive-processes and the persistence of aggressive-behavior. *Aggressive Behavior* 10(3):243-251.

Huesmann, L. R., and L. Kirwil. 2007. Why observing violence increases the risk of violent behavior in the observer. In *The Cambridge handbook of violent behavior and aggression*, edited by D. Flannery. Cambridge, UK: Cambridge University Press.

Huesmann, L. R., J. Moise-Titus, C. L. Podolski, and L. D. Eron. 2003. Longitudinal relations between children's exposure to TV violence and their aggressive and violent behavior in young adulthood: 1977-1992. *Developmental Psychology* 39(2):201-221.

Huff, D. L., and J. M. Lutz. 1974. The contagion of political unrest in independent black Africa. *Economic Geography* 50(4):352-367.

Hummer, T. A., Y. Wang, W. G. Kronenberger, K. M. Mosier, A. J. Kalnin, D. W. Dunn, and V. P. Mathews. 2010. Short-term violent video game play by adolescents alters prefrontal activity during cognitive inhibition. *Media Psychology* 13(2):136-154.

Iacoboni, M. 2008. Mirroring people: The new science of how we connect with others. New York: Farrar, Straus and Giroux.

Iacoboni, M. 2009. Imitation, empathy, and mirror neurons. In *Annual Review of Psychology*. Vol. 60. Palo Alto, CA: Annual Reviews. Pp. 653-670.

Iacoboni, M., R. P. Woods, M. Brass, H. Bekkering, J. C. Mazziotta, and G. Rizzolatti. 1999. Cortical mechanisms of human imitation. *Science* 286(5449):2526-2528.

Iacoboni, M., I. Molnar-Szakacs, V. Gallese, G. Buccino, J. C. Mazziotta, and G. Rizzolatti. 2005. Grasping the intentions of others with one's own mirror neuron system. *PLoS Biology* 3(3):e79.

Insel, B. J., and M. S. Gould. 2008. Impact of modeling on adolescent suicidal behavior. *Psychiatric Clinics of North America* 31(2):293-316.

IOM (Institute of Medicine). 1996. *Fetal alcohol syndrome: Diagnosis, epidemiology, prevention, and treatment.* Washington, DC: National Academy Press.

IOM. 2002. *Reducing suicide: A national imperative.* Washington, DC: National Academy Press.

IOM. 2009. *Preventing mental, emotional, and behavioral disorders among young people: Progress and possibilities.* Washington, DC: The National Academies Press.

Izuma, K., D. N. Saito, and N. Sadato. 2008. Processing of social and monetary rewards in the human striatum. *Neuron* 58(2):284-294.

Jacobson, C. M., and M. S. Gould. 2009. Suicide and non-suicidal self-injurious behaviors among youth: Risk and protective factors. In *Handbook of depression in adolescents*, edited by S. Nolen-Hoeksema and L. Hilt. Hillsdale, NJ: Lawrence Erlbaum Associates.

James, D. J., and L. E. Glaze. 2006. *Mental health problems of prison and jail inmates*. Washington, DC, U.S. Department of Justice, Office of Justice Programs, Bureau of Justice Statistics.

Jansen, C., C. Watts, M. Ellsberg, L. Heise, and C. Garcia-Moreno. 2004. Interviewer training in the WHO multi-country study on women's health and domestic violence. *Violence Against Women* 10(7):831-849.

Jeong, J., S. D. Shin, H. Kim, Y. C. Hong, S. S. Hwang, and E. J. Lee. 2012. The effects of celebrity suicide on copycat suicide attempt: A multi-center observational study. *Social Psychiatry and Psychiatric Epidemiology* 47(6):957-965.

Joiner, T. E. 2003. Contagion of suicidal symptoms as a function of assortative relating and shared relationship stress in college roommates. *Journal of Adolescence* 26(4):495-504.

Jones, M. C., P. Dauphinais, W. H. Sack, and P. D. Somervell. 1997. Trauma-related symptomatology among American Indian adolescents. *Journal of Traumatic Stress* 10(2):163-173.

Joshi, P. T., and D. A. O'Donnell. 2003. Consequences of child exposure to war and terrorism. *Clinical Child and Family Psychology Review* 6(4):275-292.

Kaplan, J. T., and M. Iacoboni. 2006. Getting a grip on other minds: Mirror neurons, intention understanding, and cognitive empathy. *Social Neuroscience* 1(3-4):175-183.

Kathman, J. D. 2011. Civil war diffusion and regional motivations for intervention. *Journal of Conflict Resolution* 55(6):847-876.

Kaufman, J., and E. Zigler. 1987. Do abused children become abusive parents? *American Journal of Orthopsychiatry* 57(2):186-192.

Kelly, S. 2010. The psychological consequences to adolescents of exposure to gang violence in the community: An integrated review of the literature. *Journal of Child and Adolescent Psychiatric Nursing* 23(2):61-73.

Klasen, F., G. Oettingen, J. Daniels, M. Post, C. Hoyer, and H. Adam. 2010. Posttraumatic resilience in former Ugandan child soldiers. *Child Development* 81(4):1096-1113.

Kohler, E., C. Keysers, M. A. Umilta, L. Fogassi, V. Gallese, and G. Rizzolatti. 2002. Hearing sounds, understanding actions: Action representation in mirror neurons. *Science* 297(5582):846-848.

Kokko, K., L. Pulkkinen, L. R. Huesmann, E. F. Dubow, and P. Boxer. 2009. Intensity of aggression in childhood as a predictor of different forms of adult aggression: A two-country (Finland and United States) analysis. *Journal of Research on Adolescents* 19(1):9-34.

Krug, E. G., J. A. Mercy, L. L. Dahlberg, and A. B. Zwi. 2002. The world report on violence and health. *Lancet* 360(9339):1083-1088.

Kuess, S., and R. Hatzinger. 1986. Attitudes toward suicide in the print media. *Crisis: The Journal of Crisis Intervention and Suicide Prevention* 7(2):118-125.

Landau, S. 1997. Homicide in Israel. *Homicide Studies* 1(4):377-400.

Landau, S. F. 2003. Societal costs of political violence. *Palestine-Israel Journal of Politics, Economics, and Culture* 10:28-35.

Landau, S. F., and D. Pfeffermann. 1988. A time-series analysis of violent crime and its relation to prolonged states of warfare—the Israeli case. *Criminology* 26(3):489-504.

Landau, S. F., S. D. Gvirsman, L. R. Huesmann, E. F. Dubow, P. Boxer, J. Ginges, and K. Shikaki. 2010. The effects of exposure to violence on aggressive behavior: The case of Arab and Jewish children in Israel. In *Indirect and direct aggression*, edited by K. Osterman. New York: Peter Lang.

Langan, P. A., and D. J. Levin. 2002. Recidivism of prisoners released in 1994. In *Special report/Bureau of Justice Statistics*. Washington, DC: Bureau of Justice Statistics.

Leoschut, L., and P. Burton. 2006. *Results of the 2005 National Youth Victimisation Study.* Capetown, South Africa: Centre for Justice and Crime Prevention.

Lhermitte, F., B. Pillon, and M. Serdaru. 1986. Human autonomy and the frontal lobes. Imitation and utilization behavior—a neuropsychological study of 75 patients. *Annals of Neurology* 19(4):326-334.

Li, R. P. Y., and W. R. Thompson. 1975. The "coup contagion" hypothesis. *Journal of Conflict Resolution* 19(1):63-88.

Losin, E. A., M. Iacoboni, A. Martin, and M. Dapretto. 2012. Own-gender imitation activates the brain's reward circuitry. *Social Cognitive Affective Neuroscience.*

Macdonald, G., and M. R. Leary. 2005. Why does social exclusion hurt? The relationship between social and physical pain. *Psychological Bulletin* 131(2):202-223.

Margolin, G., and E. B. Gordis. 2000. The effects of family and community violence on children. *Annual Review of Psychology* 51:445-479.

Martin, S. F. 2004. Refugee women. In *Program in migration and refugee studies.* Lanham, MD: Lexington Books.

Mathur, V. A., T. Harada, T. Lipke, and J. Y. Chiao. 2010. Neural basis of extraordinary empathy and altruistic motivation. *NeuroImage* 51(4):1468-1475.

Mendel, R. A. 2011. *No place for kids: The case for reducing juvenile incarceration.* Baltimore, MD: Annie E. Casey Foundation.

Mesoudi, A. 2009. The cultural dynamics of copycat suicide. *PLoS One* 4(9):e7252.

Michel, K., F. Conrad, T. Schlaepfer, and L. Valach. 1995. Suicide reporting in the Swiss print media. *The European Journal of Public Health* 5(3):199-203.

Miguel, E., S. M. Saiegh, and S. Satyanath. 2008. National cultures and soccer violence. *National Bureau of Economic Research Working Paper Series* No. 13968. Cambridge, MA: National Bureau of Economic Research.

Miller, G. F. 2007. Sexual selection for moral virtues. *Quarterly Review of Biology* 82(2):97-125.

Miller, K. E., and A. Rasmussen. 2010. War exposure, daily stressors, and mental health in conflict and post-conflict settings: Bridging the divide between trauma-focused and psychosocial frameworks. *Social Science & Medicine* 70(1):7-16.

Milner, J. S., C. J. Thomsen, J. L. Crouch, M. M. Rabenhorst, P. M. Martens, C. W. Dyslin, J. M. Guimond, V. A. Stander, and L. L. Merrill. 2010. Do trauma symptoms mediate the relationship between childhood physical abuse and adult child abuse risk? *Child Abuse & Neglect* 34(5):332-344.

Mitani, J. C., D. P. Watts, and S. J. Amsler. 2010. Lethal intergroup aggression leads to territorial expansion in wild chimpanzees. *Current Biology* 20(12):R507-R508.

Moffett, M. W. 2011. Ants & the art of war. *Scientific American* 305(6):84-89.

Mollica, R. 1986. *Cambodian refugee women at risk.* Washington, DC: American Psychological Association.

Morris, R. E., M. M. Anderson, and G. W. Knox. 2002. Incarcerated adolescents' experiences as perpetrators of sexual assault. *Archives of Pediatrics & Adolescent Medicine* 156(8):831-835.

Motto, J. A. 1970. Newspaper influence on suicide. *Archives of General Psychiatry* 23(2):143-148.

Mukamel, R., A. D. Ekstrom, J. Kaplan, M. Iacoboni, and I. Fried. 2010. Single-neuron responses in humans during execution and observation of actions. *Current Biology* 20(8):750-756.

Mullins, C. W., R. Wright, and B. A. Jacobs. 2004. Gender, streetlife and criminal retaliation. *Criminology* 42(4):911-940.

Murray, C. A. 2012. *Coming apart: The state of white America, 1960-2010.* 1st ed. New York: Crown Forum.

Nacos, B. L. 2009. Revisiting the contagion hypothesis: Terrorism, news coverage, and copycat attacks. *Perspectives on Terrorism* 3(3):3-14.

National Education Association. 2011. *Focus on American Indians and Alaska Natives: Bullying emerges as a contributing factor—the scourge of suicides among American Indian and Alaska Native youth.* http://www.nea.org (accessed on August 1, 2012).

Naved, R. T., and L. A. Persson. 2005. Factors associated with spousal physical violence against women in Bangladesh. *Studies in Family Planning* 36(4):289-300.

Nelson, K., and C. M. Williams. 2007. *Infectious disease epidemiology: Theory and practice.* Sudbury, MA: Jones and Bartlett Publishers.

Niederkrotenthaler, T., B. Till, N. D. Kapusta, M. Voracek, K. Dervic, and G. Sonneck. 2009. Copycat effects after media reports on suicide: A population-based ecologic study. *Social Science & Medicine* 69(7):1085-1090.

Niederkrotenthaler, T., M. Voracek, A. Herberth, B. Till, M. Strauss, E. Etzersdorfer, B. Eisenwort, and G. Sonneck. 2010. Role of media reports in completed and prevented suicide: Werther v. Papageno effects. *British Journal of Psychiatry* 197(3):234-243.

Nordstrom, B. R., Y. Gao, A. L. Glenn, M. Peskin, A. S. Rudo-Hutt, R. A. Schug, Y. L. Yang, and A. Raine. 2011. Neurocriminology. In *Aggression*, Vol. 75, edited by R. Huber, D. L. Bannasch, and P. Brennan. San Diego, CA: Elsevier Academic Press. Pp. 255-283.

Oberman, L. M., J. A. Pineda, and V. S. Ramachandran. 2007. The human mirror neuron system: A link between action observation and social skills. *Social Cognitive and Affective Neuroscience* 2(1):62-66.

Oliver, W., and C. F. Hairston. 2008. Intimate partner violence during the transition from prison to the community: Perspectives of incarcerated African American men. *Journal of Aggression, Maltreatment & Trauma* 16(3):258-276.

Osofsky, J. D. 1999. The impact of violence on children. *Future of Children* 9(3):33-49.

Panksepp, J. 1998. Affective neuroscience: The foundations of human and animal emotions. In *Series in affective science.* Oxford, UK: Oxford University Press.

Papachristos, A. V. 2009. Murder by structure: A network theory of gang homicide. *American Journal of Sociology* 115(1):74-128.

Patten, S. B., and J. A. Arboleda-Florez. 2004. Epidemic theory and group violence. *Social Psychiatry and Psychiatric Epidemiology* 39(11):853-856.

Perry, B. D. 2001. The neurodevelopmental impact of violence in childhood. In *Textbook of child and adolescent forensic psychiatry*, edited by D. Schetky and E. P. Benedek. Washington, DC: American Psychiatric Press.

Petee, T. A., K. G. Padgett, and T. S. York. 1997. Debunking the stereotype. *Homicide Studies* 1(4):317-337.

Pfeifer, J. H., M. Iacoboni, J. C. Mazziotta, and M. Dapretto. 2008. Mirroring others' emotions relates to empathy and interpersonal competence in children. *NeuroImage* 39(4):2076-2085.

Phillips, D. P. 1974. Influence of suggestion on suicide—substantive and theoretical implications of Werther effect. *American Sociological Review* 39(3):340-354.

Phillips, D. P. 1979. Suicide, motor-vehicle fatalities, and the mass-media—evidence toward a theory of suggestion. *American Journal of Sociology* 84(5):1150-1174.

Phillips, D. P., and L. L. Carstensen. 1986. Clustering of teenage suicides after television news stories about suicide. *New England Journal of Medicine* 315(11):685-689.

Phillips, D. P., K. Lesyna, and D. J. Paight. 1992. Suicide and the media. In *Assessment and prediction of suicide*, edited by R. W. Maris, et al. New York: The Guilford Press.

Pickering, M. J., and S. Garrod. 2007. Do people use language production to make predictions during comprehension? *Trends in Cognitive Science* 11(3):105-110.

Pirkis, J. E., and M. Nordentoft. 2011. Media influences on suicide and attempted suicide. In *International handbook of suicide prevention: Research, policy and practice*, edited by R. C. O'Connor, S. Platt, and J. Gordon. Oxford: Wiley-Blackwell.

Pirkis, J. E., P. M. Burgess, C. Francis, R. W. Blood, and D. J. Jolley. 2006. The relationship between media reporting of suicide and actual suicide in Australia. *Social Science & Medicine* 62(11):2874-2886.

Poijula, S., K. E. Wahlberg, and A. Dyregrov. 2001. Adolescent suicide and suicide contagion in three secondary schools. *International Journal of Emergency Mental Health* 3(3):163-168.

Popova, S., S. Lange, D. Bekmuradov, A. Mihic, and J. Rehm. 2011. Fetal alcohol spectrum disorder prevalence estimates in correctional systems: A systematic literature review. *Canadian Journal of Public Health* 102(5):336-340.

Potocky-Tripodi, M. 2002. *Best practices for social work with refugees and immigrants*. New York: Columbia University Press.

Qouta, S., and E. El Sarraj. 1992. Curfew and children's mental health. *Journal of Psychological Studies* 4:13-18.

Qouta, S., R. L. Punamki, and E. El Sarraj. 2008. Child development and family mental health in war and military violence: The Palestinian experience. *International Journal of Behavioral Development* 32(4):310-321.

Ransford, C. L., Kane, C., Slutkin, G. In press. CeaseFire: A disease control approach to reduce violence and change behavior. In *Epidemiological criminology*, edited by T. W. Akers and E. Waltermauer. London, UK: Routledge.

Rehn, F., and E. J. Sirleaf. 2002. *Women, war, peace: The independent expert's assessment on the impact of armed conflict on women and women's role in peace building*. New York: U.N. Development Fund for Women.

Reitzel-Jaffe, D., and D. A. Wolfe. 2001. Predictors of relationship abuse among young men. *Journal of Interpersonal Violence* 16(2):99-115.

Rizzolatti, G., R. Camarda, L. Fogassi, M. Gentilucci, G. Luppino, and M. Matelli. 1988. Functional organization of inferior area 6 in the macaque monkey. Area f5 and the control of distal movements. *Experimental Brain Research* 71(3):491-507.

Roberts, A. L., S. E. Gilman, G. Fitzmaurice, M. R. Decker, and K. C. Koenen. 2010. Witness of intimate partner violence in childhood and perpetration of intimate partner violence in adulthood. *Epidemiology* 21(6):809-818.

Robertson, L., K. Skegg, M. Poore, S. Williams, and B. Taylor. 2012. An adolescent suicide cluster and the possible role of electronic communication technology. *Crisis: The Journal of Crisis Intervention and Suicide Prevention*. (33)4:239-245.

Ross-Sheriff, F., R. Foy, E. Kaiser, and M. Gomes. 2012. Mental health of refugee women. In *Refugee worldwide*, edited by D. A. S. Elliot. Santa Barbara, CA: ABC-CLIO.

Rudolph, K. D., W. Troop-Gordon, and D. A. Granger. 2011. Individual differences in biological stress responses moderate the contribution of early peer victimization to subsequent depressive symptoms. *Psychopharmacology* 214(1):209-219.

Ruiz-Moreno, D., M. Pascual, M. Emch, and M. Yunus. 2010. Spatial clustering in the spatiotemporal dynamics of endemic cholera. *BMC Infectious Diseases* (10)51.

Rutter, M., H. Giller, and A. Hagell. 1998. *Antisocial behavior by young people*. Cambridge, UK: Cambridge University Press.

Sampson, R. J., S. W. Raudenbush, and F. Earls. 1997. Neighborhoods and violent crime: A multilevel study of collective efficacy. *Science* 277(5328):918-924.

Sampson, R. J., J. D. Morenoff and T. Gannon-Rowley. 2002. Assessing "neighborhood effects": Social processes and new directions in research. *Annual Review of Sociology* 28:443-478.

Sedgwick, M. 2007. Inspiration and the origins of global waves of terrorism. *Studies in Conflict & Terrorism* 30(2):97-112.

Sela-Shayovitz, R. 2005. The effects of the Second Intifada, terrorist acts, and economic changes on adolescent crime rates in Israel: A research note. *Journal of Experimental Criminology* 1(4):477-493.

Shah, A. 2010. The relationship between general population suicide rates and the Internet: A cross-national study. *Suicide and Life-Threatening Behavior* 40(2):146-150.

Shaw, C. R., and H. McKay. 1942. *Juvenile delinquency and urban areas, a study of rates of delinquents in relation to differential characteristics of local communities in American cities, Behavior Research Fund monographs*. Chicago, IL: The University of Chicago Press.

Shepherd, S. V., J. T. Klein, R. O. Deaner, and M. L. Platt. 2009. Mirroring of attention by neurons in macaque parietal cortex. *Proceedings of the National Academy of Sciences USA* 106(23):9489-9494.

Simon, H. A. 1955. A behavioral model of rational choice. *The Quarterly Journal of Economics* 69(1):99-118.

Simon, H. A. 1967. Motivational and emotional controls of cognition. *Psychological Review* 74(1):29-39.

Skogan, W., S. M. Harnett, N. Bump, and J. DuBois. 2009. *Evaluation of CeaseFire-Chicago*. Chicago, IL: Northwestern University Institute for Policy Research.

Slutkin, G., S. Okware, W. Naamara, D. Sutherland, D. Flanagan, M. Carael, E. Blas, P. Delay, and D. Tarantola. 2006. How Uganda reversed its HIV epidemic. *AIDS and Behavior* 10(4):351-360.

Soltani, A., D. Lee, and X. J. Wang. 2006. Neural mechanism for stochastic behaviour during a competitive game. *Neural Networks* 19(8):1075-1090.

Stack, S. 2003. Media coverage as a risk factor in suicide. *Journal of Epidemiology and Community Health* 57(4):238-240.

Statewide Suicide Prevention Council. 2004. *Report to the legislature 2004*. Statewide Suicide Prevention Council. http://www.hss.state.ak.us/suicideprevention/pdfs_sspc/2004sspcannualreport.pdf (accessed on August 1, 2012).

Stedman, T. L. 2012. *Stedman's medical dictionary for the health professions and nursing*. Illustrated 7th ed. Philadelphia, PA: Wolters Kluwer Health/Lippincott Williams & Wilkins.

Stein, S. 1993. *Police Board fires Burge for brutality*. Chicago Tribune, February 11.

Steiner, H., I. G. Garcia, and Z. Matthews. 1997. Posttraumatic stress disorder in incarcerated juvenile delinquents. *Journal of the American Academy of Child and Adolescent Psychiatry* 36(3):357-365.

Stevens, T. N., K. J. Ruggiero, D. G. Kilpatrick, H. S. Resnick, and B. E. Saunders. 2005. Variables differentiating singly and multiply victimized youth: Results from the National Survey of Adolescents and Implications for Secondary Prevention. *Child Maltreatment* 10(3):211-223.

Stith, S. M., K. H. Rosen, K. A. Middleton, A. L. Busch, K. Lundeberg, and R. P. Carlton. 2000. The intergenerational transmission of spouse abuse: A meta-analysis. *Journal of Marriage and the Family* 62(3):640-654.

Sue, D. W. 2010. *Microaggressions in everyday life: Race, gender, and sexual orientation*. Hoboken, NJ: Wiley.

Taylor, T. J., A. Freng, F. A. Esbensen, and D. Peterson. 2008. Youth gang membership and serious violent victimization—the importance of lifestyles and routine activities. *Journal of Interpersonal Violence* 23(10):1441-1464.

Teten, A. L., J. A. Schumacher, C. T. Taft, M. A. Stanley, T. A. Kent, S. D. Bailey, N. J. Dunn, and D. L. White. 2010. Intimate partner aggression perpetrated and sustained by male Afghanistan, Iraq, and Vietnam veterans with and without posttraumatic stress disorder. *Journal of Interpersonal Violence* 25(9):1612-1630.

Thornton, R. 1987. American Indian Holocaust and survival: A population history since 1492. 1st ed. *The civilization of the American Indian series.* Norman, OK: University of Oklahoma Press.

Toumbourou, J. W., and M. E. Gregg. 2002. Impact of an empowerment-based parent education program on the reduction of youth suicide risk factors. *Journal of Adolescent Health* 31(3):277-285.

Trafzer, C. E., J. A. Keller, and L. Sisquoc. 2006. Boarding school blues: Revisiting American Indian educational experiences. In *Indigenous education; Variation: Indigenous education.* Linclon, NE: University of Nebraska Press.

Travis, J., and M. Waul. 2003. *Prisoners once removed: The impact of incarceration and reentry on children, families, and communities.* Baltimore, MD: Urban Institute Press.

Tsfati, Y., and G. Wiemann. 2002. www.terrorism.com: Terror on the Internet. *Studies in Conflict & Terrorism* 25:317-332.

Uddin, L. Q., M. Iacoboni, C. Lange, and J. P. Keenan. 2007. The self and social cognition: The role of cortical midline structures and mirror neurons. *Trends in Cognitive Science* 11(4):153-157.

Umilta, M. A., E. Kohler, V. Gallese, L. Fogassi, L. Fadiga, C. Keysers, and G. Rizzolatti. 2001. I know what you are doing. A neurophysiological study. *Neuron* 31(1):155-165.

UNHCR (Office of the United Nations High Commissioner for Refugees). 1992. *Handbook on procedures and criteria for determining refugee status: Under the 1951 convention and the 1967 protocol relating to the status of refugees.* Geneva, Switzerland: UNHCR.

United Nations. 1993. *Declaration on the elimination of violence against women.* New York: U.N. Department of Public Information.

U.S. Conference of Mayors. 2012. *CeaseFire violence prevention model.* Paper presented at 80th Annual Meeting of the U.S. Conference of Mayors, Orlando, FL. June 15.

Veenema, A. H. 2009. Early life stress, the development of aggression and neuroendocrine and neurobiological correlates: What can we learn from animal models? *Frontal Neuroendocrinology* 30(4):497-518.

Verwimp, P. 2004. Death and survival during the 1994 genocide in Rwanda. *Population Studies (Cambridge)* 58(2):233-245.

Victoroff, J., and J. R. Adelman. 2012. Community support or contagion? A test of two theories of political violence in the Israeli-Palestinian conflict. *International Society of Political Psychology Annual Meeting,* Chicago, IL. July 7.

Victoroff, J., S. Quota, J. R. Adelman, B. Celinska, N. Stern, R. Wilcox, and R. M. Sapolsky. 2011. Support for religio-political aggression among teenaged boys in Gaza: Part II: Neuroendocrinological findings. *Aggressive Behavior* 37(2):121-132.

Waldman, R. 2005. Public health in war: Pursuing the impossible. *Harvard International Review* 27(1):60-63.

Wang, S. J., J. Modvig, and E. Montgomery. 2009. Household exposure to violence and human rights violations in western Bangladesh (I): Prevalence, risk factors and consequences. *BMC International Health and Human Rights* 9:29.

Webster, D. W., J. M. Whitehill, J. S. Vernick, and F. C. Curriero. 2012. Effects of Baltimore's Safe Streets program on gun violence: A replication of Chicago's CeaseFire program. *Journal of Urban Health.*

Whitbeck, L. B., G. W. Adams, D. R. Hoyt, and X. J. Chen. 2004. Conceptualizing and measuring historical trauma among American Indian people. *American Journal of Community Psychology* 33(3-4):119-130.

White, R. J., E. W. Gondolf, D. U. Robertson, B. J. Goodwin, and L. E. Caraveo. 2002. Extent and characteristics of woman batterers among federal inmates. *International Journal of Offender Therapy and Comparative Criminology* 46(4):412-426.

Whitlock, J. 2010. Self-injurious behavior in adolescents. *PLoS Medicine* 7(5):e1000240.

WHO (World Health Organization). 2012. *Tuberculosis fact sheet n°104*. Geneva, Switzerland: World Health Organization.

Widom, C. S. 1989. The cycle of violence. *Science* 244(4901):160-166.

Widome, R., S. M. Kehle, K. F. Carlson, M. N. Laska, A. Gulden, and K. Lust. 2011. Posttraumatic stress disorder and health risk behaviors among Afghanistan and Iraq war veterans attending college. *American Journal of Health Behavior* 35(4):387-392.

Wolf, M., G. S. van Doorn, O. Leimar, and F. J. Weissing. 2007. Life-history trade-offs favour the evolution of animal personalities. *Nature* 447(7144):581-584.

Wolff, N., and J. Shi. 2009. Contextualization of physical and sexual assault in male prisons: Incidents and their aftermath. *Journal of Correctional Health Care* 15(1):58-77; 80-82.

Wood, S. K. 2004. A woman scorned for the "least condemned" war crime: Precedent and problems with prosecuting rape as a serious crime in international criminal tribunal for Rwanda. *Columbia Journal of Gender and Law* 13:274-315.

Wright, M. 2008. Technology and terrorism: How the Internet facilitates radicalization. *Forensic Examiner* 17:14-20.

Wyman, P. A., C. H. Brown, M. LoMurray, K. Schmeelk-Cone, M. Petrova, E. Walsh, W. Wang, X. Tu, and Q. Yu. 2010. An outcome evaluation of the Sources of Strength suicide prevention program delivered by adolescent peer leaders in high schools. *American Journal of Public Health* 100(9):1653-1661.

Yellow Horse Brave Heart, M. 2003. Historical trauma response among Natives and its relationship with substance abuse: A Lakota illustration. *Journal of Psychoactive Drugs* 35(1):7-13.

Zamble, E., and F. Porporino. 1988. *Coping, behavior, and adaption in prison inmates*. New York: Springer.

Zimring, F. E., and G. Hawkins. 1997. *Crime is not the problem: Lethal violence in America*. New York: Oxford University Press.

Appendix A

Workshop Agenda

THE CONTAGION OF VIOLENCE—A WORKSHOP

APRIL 30-MAY 1, 2012

OVERVIEW:
The contagion of violence is a universal phenomenon, occurring at all levels of society and affecting a broad spectrum of individuals. This workshop will present an interdisciplinary, ecological, life-course perspective on the contagion of violence, the processes that promote it, and mechanisms to interrupt and prevent the contagion of violence and promote the contagion of nonviolence.

OBJECTIVES:
- To examine the extent of contagion of violence, the different emotional and cognitive processes through which contagion occurs, and the social and structural moderators of the contagion of violence.
- To explore the role of exposure to violence and violent victimization in the spread of interpersonal and self-directed violence and of internalizing and externalizing psychological problems.
- To understand how the contagion of violence can be interrupted and prevented and how nonviolence can become contagious.

DAY 1: MONDAY, APRIL 30, 2012

Check-in will begin at 8:15 AM. A continental breakfast will be available.

8:50 AM Welcome
PATRICK KELLEY, *Institute of Medicine*

9:00 AM Opening Remarks
VALERIE MAHOLMES, Eunice Kennedy Shriver *National Institute of Child Health & Human Development*

9:10 AM Introduction
JACQUELYN CAMPBELL, *Johns Hopkins School of Nursing and Forum on Global Violence Prevention Co-Chair*

9:20 AM Overview of the Contagion of Violence
GARY SLUTKIN, *University of Illinois at Chicago*

Moderated Q&A and Discussion

10:05 AM BREAK

10:30 AM - 12:45 PM

SESSION I: Contagion of Violence in Multiple Settings

This session will discuss how violence leads to additional violence. This can occur either as a "viral" spread of one act of violence to many acts of violence, or as a "spillover" effect from one setting or type of violence to another. How does the contagion of violence manifest across types of violence? How are types of violence interrelated? Conversely, how can the spread of violence be halted or prevented?

Facilitator: ROWELL HUESMANN, *University of Michigan*

10:30 AM Opening Remarks
ROWELL HUESMANN, *University of Michigan*

Brief Overviews

10:35 AM The Contagion of Street and Community Violence
JEFFREY FAGAN, *Columbia Law School*

10:50 AM The Contagion of Self-Directed Violence
MADELYN GOULD, *Columbia University*

11:10 AM The Contagion of Collective Violence
ERIC DUBOW, *Bowling Green State University*

11:25 AM The Contagion of Family Violence
CHARLOTTE WATTS, *London School of Hygiene and Tropical Medicine*

11:40 AM Contagion, Group Marginalization, and Resilience
CARL BELL, *Community Mental Health Council*

11:55 AM Facilitated Panel Discussion

12:20 PM Moderated Q&A and Discussion

12:45 PM - 1:45 PM LUNCH

1:45 PM - 4:00 PM

SESSION II: Theories, Processes, and Mechanisms of Contagion

How and why does violence spread? This section will explore the internal and external processes and mechanisms at work. It will also explore the interruption of such processes and mechanisms, and their use for spreading nonviolent messaging and practices. Panelists will offer a brief overview of their respective perspectives and then engage in a facilitated discussion.

Facilitator: ROBERT URSANO, *Center for the Study of Traumatic Stress*

1:45 PM Opening Remarks
ROBERT URSANO, *Center for the Study of Traumatic Stress*

Brief Overviews

1:55 PM Social-Cognitive Processes in the Contagion of Violence
ROWELL HUESMANN, *University of Michigan*

2:10 PM Social Contagion and Group Dynamics in Contagion
DEANNA WILKINSON, *The Ohio State University*

2:20 PM Contagion, Social Influence and Intimate Partner Violence
ANITA RAJ, *University California, San Diego*

2:30 PM The Role of Emotions and Evolution in Contagion
JEFFREY VICTOROFF, *University of Southern California*

2:40 PM The Neuroscience of Empathy and Contagion
JAMIL ZAKI, *Stanford University*

2:50 PM Imitation and Mirror Neurons in the Contagion Process
MARCO IACOBONI, *University of California, Los Angeles*

3:00 PM Facilitated Panel Discussion

3:35 PM Moderated Q&A and Discussion

3:50 PM Wrap-Up
ROBERT URSANO, *Center for the Study of Traumatic Stress*

4:00 PM BREAK

4:20 PM - 5:30 PM

SESSION III: The Contagion at Work

This session will explore some recent, real-world examples of the spread of violence from singular events or settings. Speakers will also examine possibilities for preventing violence or mitigating the effects of violence.

Facilitator: GARY SLUTKIN, *University of Illinois at Chicago*

4:20 PM Opening Remarks
GARY SLUTKIN, *University of Illinois at Chicago*

4:25 PM Contagion in the London Riots
JASON FEATHERSTONE, *Surviving Our Streets*

4:40 PM Contagion in the Arab Spring
ZAINAB AL-SUWAIJ, *American Islamic Congress*

4:55 PM   Facilitated Panel Discussion and Moderated Q&A

5:30 PM   ADJOURN DAY 1

DAY 2: TUESDAY, MAY 1, 2012

Check-in will begin at 8:15 AM. A continental breakfast will be available.

9:00 AM   Overview of Day 1
ROWELL HUESMANN, *University of Michigan*

9:20 AM - 11:30 AM

SESSION IV: Social and Structural Moderators/Cofactors of the Contagion of Violence

This session will focus on how systems and practices can contribute to the exacerbation of, or the reduction and prevention of, the transmission of violence. Panelists will offer a brief overview of their respective perspectives and then engage in a facilitated discussion.

Facilitator: EVELYN P. TOMASZEWSKI, *National Association of Social Workers*

9:20 AM   Opening Remarks
EVELYN P. TOMASZEWSKI, *National Association of Social Workers*

Brief Overviews

9:30 AM   The Role of Punishment, Incarceration, and Re-entry
BARRY KRISBERG, *University of California, Berkeley, School of Law*

9:45 AM   The Role of Historical Trauma
IRIS PRETTYPAINT, *Native Aspirations, Kauffman & Associates, Inc.*

10:00 AM   The Role of Family and Positive Parenting
DEBORAH GORMAN-SMITH, *Chapin Hall*

10:15 AM   The Role of Migration and Population Displacement
FARIYAL ROSS-SHERIFF, *Howard University*

10:30 AM Facilitated Panel Discussion

11:00 AM Audience Discussion and Moderated Q&A

11:30 AM BREAK and LUNCH (*provided*)

11:50 AM - 2:00 PM

SESSION V: Film Screening: *The Interrupters*

Shot over the course of a year, *The Interrupters* captures a period in Chicago when it became a national symbol for the violence in American cities. *The Interrupters* tells the stories of three Violence Interrupters who work for an innovative organization, CeaseFire, which uses a public health model to stop the cycle of violence in neighborhoods and communities. The Violence Interrupters, who have credibility because of their own personal histories, intervene in conflicts before they explode into violence.
Note: This film contains scenes of violence and adult language.

11:50 AM Overview
    BRIAN FLYNN, *Uniformed Services University School of Medicine*

12:10 PM Screening

2:15 PM BREAK

2:35 PM - 3:10 PM

SECTION VI: Scaling Up or Translating Programs
to Interrupt the Contagion of Violence

Following the film, a panel of speakers will share experiences with interruption in various settings, from the community to health care settings to elsewhere. Speakers will offer thoughts on how violence can be interrupted, and how programs using the interruption mechanism can be scaled up or translated.

Facilitators:
BRIAN FLYNN, *Uniformed Services University School of Medicine*
CHARLOTTE WATTS, *London School of Hygiene and Tropical Medicine*

2:35 PM Overview
CHARLOTTE WATTS, *London School of Hygiene and Tropical Medicine*

2:40 PM Panel

The Experience of Interruption
TIO HARDIMAN, *CeaseFire Illinois*

School-Based Violence and Interruption
PATRICK BURTON, *Center for Justice and Crime Prevention, South Africa*

Hospitals and Interruption
JOHN A. RICH, *Drexel University, Center for Nonviolence and Social Justice*

Interrupting Family Violence
VALERIE MAHOLMES, Eunice Kennedy Shriver *National Institute of Child Health & Human Development*

3:10 PM Facilitated Panel Discussion

3:30 PM Moderated Q&A

4:00 PM ADJOURN DAY 2

Appendix B

Glossary

Agent: factor whose presence (or absence) is necessary for the occurrence of a disease.

Carrier: individual who harbors a specific infectious agent without visible symptoms of the disease. In the case of violence, a carrier can transmit violence without directly committing an act of violence.

Cluster: aggregation of cases of a disease that are closely grouped in time and place. Frequently the expected number of cases is not known.

Contagion: transmission of a disease from one individual to another through direct contact or indirect exposure.

Disease: condition in which the functioning of the body or a part of the body is interfered with or damaged. Usually the body will show some signs and symptoms of the interference with or damaged functioning and exhibit adverse health outcomes. A disease, such as violence, can be either acute or chronic.

> *Infectious disease:* disease that is caused by the invasion of a host by agents and can be transmitted to other individuals.

Epidemic: occurrence of cases of a disease in a community or region that is in excess of the number of cases normally expected for that disease in that area at that time.

Exposure: instance of being subjected to an action or influence.

> *Dose exposure:* refers to the amount of exposure, which can be along spectrum of acute to chronic.

Host: individual in which a disease lives.

Immunity: resistance to infection; in the case of violence, an individual's level of immunity is frequently increased through exposure to protective factors and decreased through exposure to risk factors.

Incubation: period of inapparent infection following disease exposure and ending with the onset of symptoms of apparent infection. In the case of violence, the incubation period varies widely; individuals can be exposed to violence, but not exhibit any violent behavior until a significant period of time has lapsed.

Infection: entry and development of an infectious agent in the body. An infection can be either apparent (showing outward symptoms of illness) or unapparent (showing no outward symptoms of illness).

Interruption: prevention of disease transmission.

Latency: time period between infection and infectivity to others.

Mediators and cofactor: either a risk or protective factor that affects the transmission or prevention and interruption of a disease.

Protective factor: aspect of personal behavior or lifestyle, an environmental exposure, or an inborn or inherited characteristic that is associated with a decreased occurrence of disease.

Risk factor: aspect of personal behavior or lifestyle, an environmental exposure, or an inborn or inherited characteristic that is associated with an increased occurrence of disease.

Spread: movement of an infectious disease from a vector to a host. In the case of violence, one type of violence can spread virally to multiple cases of the same type of violence, such as suicide clusters. Violence also can spread through a spillover effect, with one type of violence spreading to other types; for example, child abuse can lead to later occurrences of intimate partner violence.

Susceptibility: level of immunity or resistance to a disease. Susceptibility varies depending on mediators and cofactors such as time, context, and biological circumstances.

Transmission: any mechanism by which an infectious disease is spread from a source to an individual. Violence can be transmitted horizontally, from individual to individual, and vertically, through intergenerational transmission.

Vector: carrier that transmits an infectious agent from one host to another.

Appendix C

Speaker Biographical Sketches

Zainab Al-Suwaij is a co-founder of the American Islamic Congress (AIC) and has been its executive director since its inception in 2001. In the wake of the 9/11 terror attacks, Ms. Al-Suwaij left her teaching position at Yale University to launch AIC with the mission of building interfaith and inter-ethnic understanding and to represent the diversity of American Muslim life. Over the past decade, Ms. Al-Suwaij's leadership has expanded AIC into an international organization with bureaus worldwide, including the United States, Egypt, Iraq, and its newest location, Tunisia. Under her direction, AIC has trained hundreds of young Middle Eastern activists in the methods of nonviolent protest and social media mobilization, empowering them to take on regimes during the Arab Spring. In Iraq, she launched a program that disrupts and mediates tribal and sectarian violence as it happens, saving dozens of lives in Basra and Baghdad. Ms. Al-Suwaij's vision for acceptance and understanding in the United States is being realized through AIC's growing campus initiative, Project Nur, as well as its Interfaith Councils and groundbreaking Witness Series. Ms. Al-Suwaij is an outspoken advocate for women's equality, civil rights, and interfaith understanding. She has briefed Congress and the White House and has been invited to speak at numerous panel events, universities, and think tanks. Ms. Al-Suwaij has published editorials in the three largest American newspapers: *New York Times*, *Wall Street Journal*, and *USA Today*. She has appeared on NPR, BBC, Al-Jazeera, CBS, ABC, MSNBC, CNN, and Fox. Named an "Ambassador of Peace" by the Interreligious and International Peace Council, Ms. Al-Suwaij has received Dialogue on Diversity's Liberty Award and was recognized as "2006 International Person of the Year" by the National Liberty Museum. Raised in Basra, Iraq, Ms. Al-Suwaij fled the country after participating in the 1991 uprising against Saddam Hussein and is now a U.S. citizen living in the Washington, DC, area.

Carl C. Bell, M.D., a clinical professor of psychiatry and public health, is the director of the Institute for Juvenile Research (IJR) at the University of Illinois at Chicago (UIC). IJR is a century-old, multimillion-dollar academic institute providing child and family research, training, and service, employing 257 academic faculty and support staff. Dr. Bell is also the president and chief executive (CEO) of Community Mental Health Council & Foundation, Inc., in Chicago, a large multimillion dollar comprehensive community mental health center employing 390 social service experts. Over 40 years, he has published more than 450 articles, chapters, and books on mental health and authored *The Sanity of Survival*. He has been interviewed by *Ebony*, *Jet*, *Essence*, *Emerge*, *New York Times*, *Chicago Tribune Magazine*, *People Magazine*, *Chicago Reporter*, *Nightline*, *ABC News*, National Public Radio, *CBS Sunday Morning*, the *News Hour with Jim Lehrer*, the *Tom Joyner Morning Show*, *Chicago Tonight*, and the *Today* show. A graduate of UIC, he earned his M.D. from Meharry College in Nashville. In 2011, Dr. Bell received the American Psychiatric Association's annual Solomon Carter Fuller Award at Institute on Psychiatric Services. He completed his psychiatric residency in 1974 at the Illinois State Psychiatric Institute/IJR in Chicago.

Patrick Burton, M.Sc., H.Dip., is the executive director of the Centre for Justice and Crime Prevention (CJCP), a Cape Town–based nongovernmental organization engaged in the field of social justice and crime prevention, with a particular focus on children and youth. He has undertaken work in the security; HIV/AIDS and health; information and communications technology; and small business sectors. He previously worked for the National Department of Provincial and Local Government, as well as to the National Department of Communications. While at CJCP, Mr. Burton has worked on the first national youth victimization study to be conducted in South Africa, youth resilience to violence study, a national school violence baseline study, and a cyber-violence pilot study. Other more recent projects undertaken include explorations into the causes and nature of youth violence, and intensive work into the extent and nature of school violence in South Africa and the region. He has undertaken work in Bangladesh, the Democratic Republic of Congo, Ethiopia, India, Malawi, Mozambique, Namibia, South Africa, South Sudan, and Tanzania. Mr. Burton is a postgraduate development researcher, having graduated from the University of the Witwatersrand with a higher diploma in development planning, and from the University of KwaZulu-Natal (Durban) with an M.S. in development studies, with a gender focus.

Jacquelyn C. Campbell, Ph.D., R.N. (*Planning Committee Member*), is the Anna D. Wolf chair and professor at the Johns Hopkins University (JHU) School of Nursing, with a joint appointment in the Bloomberg School of Public Health and one of the inaugural Gilman Scholars at JHU. She is also the national program director of the Robert Wood Johnson Foundation Nurse Faculty Scholars program. Dr. Campbell has been conducting advocacy policy work and research in the area of violence against women since 1980, with 12 major federally funded research grants and more than 220 articles and 7 books. She is an elected member of the Institute of Medicine (IOM) of the National Academy of Sciences (NAS), and the American Academy of Nursing as well as chair of the Board of Directors of Futures without Violence. She served on the Department of Defense (DoD) Task Force on Domestic Violence and has provided consultation to the Department of Health and Human Services (HHS), Centers for Disease Control and Prevention (CDC), World Health Organization (WHO), and U.S. Agency for International Development, She received the National Friends of the National Institute of Nursing Research Research Pathfinder Award, the Sigma Theta Tau International Nurse Researcher Award, and the American Society of Criminology Vollmer Award for advancing justice. Dr. Campbell co-chaired the Steering Committee for the WHO multi-country study on Violence Against Women and Women's Health. She has been appointed to three IOM/NAS Committees evaluating evidence in various aspects the area of violence against women, and currently serves on the IOM Board on Global Health and co-chairs the IOM Forum on Global Violence Prevention. She is also a member of the Fulbright Specialist Roster and does work in collaboration with shelters, governments, criminal justice agencies, schools of nursing, and health care settings in countries such as Australia, the Democratic Republic of the Congo, Haiti, New Zealand, South Africa, and Spain.

Eric F. Dubow, Ph.D., is professor of clinical and developmental psychology at Bowling Green State University and an adjunct research scientist at the University of Michigan's Institute for Social Research. His research and writings on stress and coping in adolescents were some of the first to illuminate the role that the child's coping and family and community resources play in promoting resilience, while his longitudinal research on the development of aggression has demonstrated the long-term detrimental consequences of early aggressiveness in youth. His recent longitudinal studies of Palestinian and Israeli youth have shown how war violence promotes both interpersonal violence and posttraumatic stress symptoms in youth exposed to the war violence. Professor Dubow is currently associate editor of *Developmental Psychology* and bulletin editor for the International Society for Research on Aggression. He also participates on National Institutes of

Health (NIH) review panels for risk and protective factors. He is a member of the American Psychological Association, Society for Research in Child Development, Society for Research on Adolescence, and International Society for Research on Aggression. He obtained his undergraduate degree at Columbia University and his Ph.D. at UIC.

Jeffrey Fagan, Ph.D., is the Isidor and Seville Sulzbacher Professor of Law and professor of epidemiology at Columbia University, and director of the Center for Crime, Community and Law at Columbia Law School. He also is a senior scholar at Yale Law School. His research and scholarship examines policing, the legitimacy of the criminal law, capital punishment, legal socialization of adolescents, neighborhoods and crime, and juvenile crime and punishment. He served on the Committee on Law and Justice of the NAS from 2000 to 2006. From 1996 to 2006, he was a member of the MacArthur Foundation's Research Network on Adolescent Development and Juvenile Justice. He is a founding member of the National Consortium on Violence Research, the Working Group on Legitimacy and the Criminal Law of the Russell Sage Foundation, and the Working Group on Incarceration at Russell Sage. From 2002 to 2005, he was a Robert Wood Johnson Foundation Health Policy Research Fellow. He is past editor of the *Journal of Research in Crime and Delinquency*, and serves on the editorial boards of several journals on criminology and law. He is a fellow of the American Society of Criminology.

Jason Featherstone, director for Surviving Our Streets, director of Violence Prevention with The Safety Box, and lead founder for the Chaos Theory organization, is committed to the reduction of street-related violence in the United Kingdom. Born to Guyanese parents in 1979, Featherstone's first home from the hospital was a squat on the Woodberry Down estate, north London, moving shortly thereafter to a flat in Tottenham. Making the transition from victim to offender to practitioner, he has a grounded insight into the world to which so many of our young people succumb. Having grown up in Tottenham, the area that was the focal point for the UK 2011 riots, he experienced many of the issues facing the youth of today in inner-city London. Unfortunately these experiences included the loss of a number of friends and a cousin to gun and knife violence. The recent London riots hit very close to home for Featherstone. The footage of Allied Carpets, a local landmark, burning to the ground, was a stark reminder of the tensions that exist in Tottenham and indeed throughout the most deprived areas in London. Once the violence took root, the transmission from area to area, inclusive of neighboring communities with gang rivalries, was swift and fierce. In 2008 he received a commendation from the Home Office Violent Crime Directorate. He was selected for the pioneering Bravehearts program, a Home Office initiative. As 1 of 12 youth leaders selected to take part in the weeklong development program in the Scottish Black Isles, he was pushed to his limits in the survival setting and tasked with conceptualizing new responses to knife and gun violence.

Brian W. Flynn, Ed.D., M.A. (*Planning Committee Member*) is a consultant, writer, trainer, and speaker specializing in preparation for, response to, and recovery from, the psychosocial aspects of large-scale emergencies and disasters. He has served numerous national and international organizations, states, and academic institutions. In addition, he currently serves as associate director of the Center for the Study of Traumatic Stress, and adjunct professor of psychiatry, department of psychiatry, Uniformed Services University of Health Sciences, in Bethesda, Maryland. In 2002, he left federal service as a rear admiral/assistant surgeon general in the U.S. Public Health Service. He has directly operated, and supervised the operation of, the federal government's domestic disaster mental health program (including terrorism), programs in suicide and youth violence prevention, child trauma, refugee mental health, women's and minority mental health concerns, and rural mental health. He has served as an advisor to many federal departments and agencies, states, and national professional organizations. He is recognized internationally for his expertise in large-scale trauma and has served as an advisor to practitioners, academicians, and government officials in many nations. He received his B.A. from North Carolina Wesleyan College, his M.A. in clinical psychology from East Carolina University, and his Ed.D. in mental health administration from the University of Massachusetts at Amherst.

Deborah Gorman-Smith, Ph.D., is a senior research fellow at Chapin Hall and principal investigator and director of the Chicago Center for Youth Violence Prevention, 1 of 10 National Academic Centers of Excellence funded by the CDC. Her program of research, grounded in a public health perspective, is focused on advancing knowledge about development, risk, and prevention of aggression and violence, with specific focus on minority youth living in poor urban settings. Dr. Gorman-Smith has been or is now is principal or co–principal investigator on several longitudinal risk and prevention intervention studies funded by the *Eunice Kennedy Shriver* National Institute of Child Health & Human Development (NICHD), National Institute on Drug Abuse, CDC, Substance Abuse and Mental Health Services Administration (SAMHSA), and the W.T. Grant Foundation. Dr. Gorman-Smith has published extensively in areas related to youth violence, including the relationships among community characteristics, family functioning, and aggression and violence, including partner violence, and the impact of family-focused preventive interventions. She also serves as senior research fellow with the Coalition for Evidence Based Policy, a nonprofit, nonpartisan organization whose mission is to promote government policy based on rigorous evidence of program effectiveness. She currently serves on the board of directors for the Society for Prevention Research, in addition to her service on other national, state, and university committees. She served as a visiting scholar at the Joint Center for Poverty Research at Northwestern University/University of Chicago. Dr. Gorman-Smith received her Ph.D. in clinical-developmental psychology at UIC.

Madelyn Gould, Ph.D., M.P.H., is a professor in psychiatry and epidemiology, and deputy director of research training in child psychiatry at Columbia University. Dr. Gould's research interests include the epidemiology of youth suicide and the evaluation of suicide prevention interventions across the age span. Her participation in U.S. national government commissions includes the 1978 President's Commission on Mental Health, the 1989 Secretary of HHS's Task Force on Youth Suicide, and the Surgeon General's 1999 National Suicide Prevention Strategy. She contributed to the CDC's community response plan for suicide clusters (1988) and recommendations to optimize media reporting of suicide (1994), and more recently contributed to www.reportingonmedia.org. The recipient of the Shneidman Award for Research from the American Association of Suicidology in 1991, the New York State Office of Mental Health Research Award in 2002, the American Foundation for Suicide Prevention Research Award in 2006, and the New York State Suicide Prevention Center's Excellence in Suicide Prevention Award in 2011, Dr. Gould has a strong commitment to applying her research to program and policy development.

Tio Hardiman, M.A., director for CeaseFire Illinois and creator of the Violence Interrupter Initiative, has dedicated his life and career to community organizing for peace and social change. In 1999, Mr. Hardiman joined CeaseFire, an award-winning public health model that has been scientifically proven to reduce shootings and killings. In 2008, under Mr. Hardiman's direction, CeaseFire received additional funding from the State of Illinois to immediately expand from 5 to 15 communities and from 20 to 130 Outreach Workers and Violence Interrupters. Today, CeaseFire has been replicated in 15 Chicago communities, 7 cities in Illinois, 15 cities nationwide, England, Iraq, and South Africa. In addition, more than 30 cities and 20 nations concerned about their own levels of shootings and killings have expressed interest in learning more about the model. *The Interrupters* documentary based on Mr. Hardiman's work has won film festivals across the nation. *The Interrupters* was released in theaters across the nation in 2011. Growing up in Chicago's notorious Henry Horner Housing Projects, Mr. Hardiman witnessed firsthand the devastating effect the violence epidemic has on a community. From that early exposure, he committed himself to ending violence in Chicago. Before joining CeaseFire, Mr. Hardiman organized more than 100 block clubs to strategize community plans for public safety on behalf of the Chicago Alliance for Neighborhood Safety and held leadership positions for Bethel New Life and Chicago's CAPS Program. He holds a bachelor's degree in liberal arts from Northeastern University and a master's degree in inner city studies.

L. Rowell Huesmann, Ph.D., M.S. (*Planning Committee Chair*), is the Amos N. Tversky Collegiate Professor of Psychology and Communication Studies and director of the Research Center for Group Dynamics at the University of Michigan's Institute for Social Research. He is also editor of the journal *Aggressive Behavior* and past president of the International Society for Research on Aggression. His research over the past 40 years has focused on the psychological foundations of aggressive and violent behavior and on how predisposing personal factors interact with precipitating situational factors to engender violent behavior. This research has included several life span longitudinal studies showing how the roots of aggressive behavior are often established in childhood. One particular interest has been investigating how children learn through imitation and how children's exposure to violence in the family, schools, community, and mass media stimulates the development of their own aggressive and violent behavior over time. He has conducted longitudinal studies on the effects of exposure to violence at multiple sites in the United States as well as in Finland, Israel, Palestine, and Poland. These studies have shown that simply seeing a lot of violence (political violence, family violence, community violence, media violence) in childhood changes children's thinking and perceptions, and increases the risk of interpersonal aggressive behavior later in life. He has also conducted research showing that interventions that change children's beliefs about the appropriateness of conflict and aggression can be effective in preventing aggression. In 2005, Dr. Huesmann was the recipient of the American Psychological Association's award for Distinguished Lifetime Contributions to Media Psychology.

Marco Iacoboni, M.D., Ph.D., is a neurologist and neuroscientist originally from Italy. Currently, he is professor of psychiatry and biobehavioral sciences at the David Geffen School of Medicine at University of California, Los Angeles, and director of the Transcranial Magnetic Stimulation laboratory of the Ahmanson-Lovelace Brain Mapping Center. Dr. Iacoboni investigates the neural basis of sensory-motor integration, imitation, and social learning. In particular, Dr. Iacoboni pioneered the research on the human mirror neuron system and its role in social behavior and learning, and its disorders. Dr. Iacoboni's research has been funded by the NIH and the

National Science Foundation. He describes the research on mirror neurons for the general reader in his recent book *Mirroring People: The Science of Empathy and How We Connect with Others.*

Patrick W. Kelley, M.D., Dr.P.H., joined the IOM in 2003 as the director of the Board on Global Health. He has subsequently also been appointed the director of the Board on African Science Academy Development. Dr. Kelley has overseen a portfolio of IOM expert consensus studies and convening activities on subjects as wide ranging as the evaluation of the U.S. emergency plan for international AIDS relief (PEPFAR); the U.S. commitment to global health; sustainable surveillance for zoonotic infections; cardiovascular disease prevention in low- and middle-income countries; interpersonal violence prevention in low- and middle-income countries; and microbial threats to health. He also directs a unique capacity-building effort, the African Science Academy Development Initiative, which over 10 years aims to strengthen the capacity of eight African academies to provide independent, evidence-based advice to their governments on scientific matters. Prior to coming to the NAS, Dr. Kelley served in the U.S. Army for more than 23 years as a physician, residency director, epidemiologist, and program manager. In his last DoD position, Dr. Kelley founded and directed the DoD Global Emerging Infections Surveillance and Response System. This responsibility entailed managing surveillance and capacity-building partnerships with numerous elements of the federal government and with health ministries in over 45 developing countries. He also founded the DoD Accession Medical Standards Analysis and Research Activity. Dr. Kelley is an experienced communicator having lectured in English or Spanish in more than 20 countries. He has published more than 65 scholarly papers, book chapters, and monographs. Dr. Kelley obtained his M.D. from the University of Virginia and his Dr.P.H. in epidemiology from the Johns Hopkins School of Hygiene and Public Health. He is also board-certified in preventive medicine and public health.

Barry A. Krisberg, Ph.D., is the research and policy director of the Chief Justice Earl Warren Institute on Law and Social Policy at the University of California, Berkeley, Law School. He is also a lecturer in residence in the Juris Doctor Program at Berkeley Law and was recently a visiting scholar at John Jay College in New York City. He is known nationally for his research and expertise on juvenile justice issues and is often called on as a resource for professionals, foundations, and the media. Dr. Krisberg was appointed by the legislature to serve on the California Blue Ribbon Commission on Inmate Population Management. He has served on almost all major statewide task forces on California corrections issues over the past 20 years. He is past president and fellow of the Western Society of Criminology and was the chair of the California Attorney General's Research Advisory

Committee. In 1993 he was the recipient of the August Vollmer Award, the American Society of Criminology's most prestigious award. The Jessie Ball duPont Fund named him the 1999 Grantee of the Year for his outstanding commitment and expertise in the area of juvenile justice and delinquency prevention. In 2009, he received special recognition by the Annie E. Casey Foundation for his contributions to the Juvenile Detention Alternatives Initiative. Dr. Krisberg was appointed to chair an Expert Panel to investigate the conditions in the California youth prisons. In 2004, he was named in a consent decree to help develop remedial plans and to monitor many of the mandated reforms in the California Division of Juvenile Justice. He has also assisted the Special Litigation Branch of the U.S. Department of Justice (DOJ) on Civil Rights of Institutionalized Persons Act investigations. He has been retained by the New York State Office of Children and Family Services to assist in juvenile justice reforms. Dr. Krisberg received his master's degree in criminology and a doctorate in sociology, both from the University of Pennsylvania.

Valerie Maholmes, Ph.D., is the program director for the Child and Family Processes/Maltreatment and Violence Research Program in the Child Development and Behavior Branch at the NICHD. In this capacity she provides scientific leadership on research and research training relevant to normative development in children from the newborn period through adolescence, and on the impact of specific aspects of physical and social environments on the health and psychological development of infants, children, and adolescents. Specifically, she supports research that addresses the public health, justice, social services, and educational problems associated with childhood and adolescent exposure to violence, as well as studies examining the trajectories that may lead to antisocial behavior, conduct problems, and aggression. In addition, Dr. Maholmes' program includes a focus on the antecedents and consequences of child abuse and neglect as well as psychosocial and psychobiological factors that shed light on the mechanisms by which child abuse and neglect result in harmful effects. A goal of her program is to support the development theory-driven prevention and intervention approaches that reduce the risk for maltreatment and ameliorate its effects on child development. More recently, Dr. Maholmes initiated a funding opportunity calling for research on children in military families to examine whether there are long-term consequences of military deployment and reintegration on child and family functioning. She serves on several federal interagency working groups addressing crosscutting issues related to child and adolescent development, vulnerable children in low- to middle-income countries, teen data violence, bullying, and behavioral and social sciences research. She is currently the co-chair of the NIH Child Abuse and Neglect Working Group. Before joining the NICHD, Dr. Maholmes was a faculty member at the

Yale Child Study Center where she served in numerous capacities, including director of research and policy for the School Development Program, and was named the Irving B. Harris assistant professor of child psychiatry. In 2003, Dr. Maholmes was awarded the Executive Branch Science Policy Fellowship sponsored by the Society for Research in Child Development and the American Association for the Advancement of Science.

Iris PrettyPaint, Ph.D., is the Native Aspirations project director at Kauffman & Associates, Inc., headquartered in Spokane, Washington. Native Aspirations is funded by SAMHSA to provide national training and technical assistance to 65 American Indian and Alaskan Native villages to reduce violence, bullying, and suicide among youth. The Native Aspirations project contributes to a nationwide tribal movement toward healing, violence prevention, and positive youth development. Dr. PrettyPaint provides administrative oversight for an 11-member team to conduct data-driven community prevention planning, build community coalitions, and the implement evidence, practice, and culture-based interventions. Dr. PrettyPaint has more than 30 years of experience as an educator, researcher, and evaluator. She is a leading authority on cultural resilience, student retention, and indigenous evaluation, and her publications address issues of traditional native culture and resilience, family support models, cultural and school partnerships, and indigenous theoretical foundations on educational persistence. She has delivered training and technical assistance on a variety of topics, such as historical trauma, bullying, cultural resilience, youth leadership, substance abuse, post-vention, curriculum development, indigenous research methods, student retention, and sustainability.

Anita Raj, Ph.D., is a professor in the division of global public health, department of medicine and a senior fellow in the Center for Global Justice at the University of California, San Diego, as well as an adjunct professor of medicine at Boston University. Trained as a developmental psychologist, she has 20 years of experience conducting research on sexual and reproductive health/HIV/sexually transmitted infections, gender-based violence and inequities, substance misuse and abuse, and the intersection of these issues. Her current research is based in North America, Russia, and South Asia. This work includes qualitative and quantitative research to support intervention development and implementation, as well as efficacy and effectiveness trials to evaluate behavioral interventions. Dr. Raj has served as principal investigator or co-principal investigator on more than 30 grants from various federal funding agencies, including the NIH, CDC, SAMHSA, Office of Minority Health, and Packard Foundation; she has authored or co-authored more than 100 peer-reviewed publications from these efforts. Her research on gender-based violence has focused on culturally specific and contextual vulnerabilities to violence among vulnerable populations for women. She has published research on the intersection of immigration-related abuse (e.g., threats of deportation, withholding of documentation papers) with spousal violence against immigrant women in the United States, as well as the role of immigration laws in reinforcing this intersection. This work was used to support change of the Violence Against Women Act to support better protections for non-U.S.-born victims of gender-based violence, including the development of the U-Visa, which protects women victims who were in the United States on spousal dependent visas. Over the past 5 years, Dr. Raj has focused her research on understanding girl child marriage (marriage prior to age 18), its intersection with gender-based violence, and its impact on maternal and child health globally. She has been working with various international organizations (e.g., the Elders and Girls Not Brides, UNICEF) to increase recognition of this issue as a global public health concern disproportionately affecting sub-Saharan Africa and South Asia and contributing to issues of HIV and maternal and infant mortality in these regions. In addition to her research, Dr. Raj has for the past 20 years been involved with various governmental committees and nongovernmental and community-based organizations working and advocating for immigrant rights, gender equity and violence prevention, and reproductive rights.

John A. Rich, M.D., M.P.H., is professor and chair of health management and policy at the Drexel University School of Public Health. He has been a leader in the field of public health, and his work has focused on serving one of the nation's most ignored and underserved populations— African-American men in urban settings. In 2006, Dr. Rich was granted a MacArthur Foundation Fellowship. In awarding this distinction, the Foundation cited his work to design "new models of health care that stretch across the boundaries of public health, education, social service, and justice systems to engage young men in caring for themselves and their peers." Prior to Drexel University, Dr. Rich served as the medical director of the Boston Public Health Commission. As a primary care doctor at Boston Medical Center, Dr. Rich created the Young Men's Health Clinic and initiated the Boston HealthCREW, a program to train inner city young men to become peer health educators who focus on the health of men and boys in their communities. In 2009, Dr. Rich was inducted into the IOM. His recently published book about urban violence, *Wrong Place, Wrong Time: Trauma and Violence in the Lives of Young Black Men,* has drawn critical acclaim. He earned his Dartmouth A.B. degree in English, his M.D. from Duke University Medical School, and his M.P.H. from the Harvard School of Public Health. He completed his internship and residency at the Massachusetts General Hospital and was a fellow in general internal medicine at

Harvard Medical School. He received an honorary doctor of science degree from Dartmouth in 2007 and now serves on its board of trustees.

Fariyal Ross-Sheriff, Ph.D., is a graduate professor and the director of Ph.D. program in social work at Howard University. Her area of specialization is displaced populations. These populations include two major groups—internationally: refugees, immigrants, and undocumented migrants, and within the United States: the homeless and disaster victims. Within displaced populations Dr. Ross-Sheriff's work emphasizes women, children, and the elderly. Dr. Ross-Sheriff has worked extensively with Muslim refugees in Pakistan to examine the challenges facing refugees and service providers, and in Afghanistan to facilitate the repatriation and resettlement of refugees. In addition, she has conducted research on the role of women in the repatriation process. She has conducted training for service providers and made several presentations at conferences on refugee issues in countries of first asylum and different aspects of adaptation of refugees and immigrants to the United States. She serves as the editor in chief for *Affilia: Journal of Women and Social Work*, and a member on the editorial boards of *Social Thought, Affilia, Journal of Immigrant and Refugee Services*, and *Social Development Issues*. Among her many publication are articles on women issues; two co-edited books, *Mental Health and People of Color: Curriculum Development and Change*, Howard University Press, 1983, and *Social Work Practice with Asian Americans*, Sage Publications, Inc., 1992; and a co-authored monograph titled *Muslim Refugees in the United States*. Her current research focuses on transnational research on women in post-war situations and living in ultra-poverty. With Dr. R.A. English, she has developed the M.S.W. degree–level specialization in social work with displaced populations. She has taught in this specialization area for more than 20 years.

Gary Slutkin, M.D. (*Planning Committee Member*), is a physician and epidemiologist, an innovator in violence reduction, and the founder/executive director of Cure Violence (formerly known as CeaseFire), a scientifically proven, health approach to violence reduction using disease control methods. Cure Violence has now been statistically validated to reduce shootings and killings by two independent evaluations conducted by the DOJ and CDC, respectively, in multiple communities in Chicago and Baltimore. Dr. Slutkin applied lessons learned from more than a decade fighting epidemics in Africa and Asia to the creation of a public health model to reduce violence through behavior change and disease control methods. He is an Ashoka Fellow, a professor of epidemiology and international health at the University of Illinois at Chicago, a senior advisor to the WHO, and the 2009 winner of the Search for a Common Ground Award. Dr. Slutkin received his M.D. from the University of Chicago Pritzker School of Medicine, and did his internship and residency at San Francisco General Hospital (SFGH). He served as chief resident at SFGH and did his infectious disease fellowship there. He then became director of the Tuberculosis Control for the City of San Francisco (1981-1985), where he learned infectious disease control methods, and then moved to Somalia to work on tuberculosis, cholera and as counterpart to the National Director of Primary Health Care Program for Somalia (1985-1987). He then worked for the World Health Organization (1987-1994) reversing epidemics, including being principally responsible for supporting Uganda's AIDS program—the only country to have reversed its AIDS epidemic. Dr. Slutkin was also responsible for setting up the HIV sentinel surveillance system for monitoring country and global trends in HIV, running the intervention development unit at WHO, and setting up the country programs for the 13 countries in the epicenter of the AIDS epidemic for the WHO Global Program on AIDS. Dr. Slutkin's work was featured in Studs Terkel's *Will the Circle Be Unbroken*, profiled in *Blocking the Transmission*, a New York Magazine cover story by bestselling author Alex Kotlowitz, and represented in the award-winning documentary *The Interrupters*.

Evelyn P. Tomaszewski, M.S.W. (*Planning Committee Member*), is a senior policy advisor within the Human Rights and International Affairs Division of the National Association of Social Workers (NASW), where she directs the NASW HIV/AIDS Spectrum Project. The project is a multiphase, federally funded project based on a training of trainer model that develops provider capacity—through training, education, and technical assistance—to better address the clinical practice and policy issues relevant to the range of health and behavioral health issues of living with HIV/AIDS and co-occurring chronic illnesses. Ms. Tomaszewski promotes the NASW Global HIV/AIDS Initiative in collaboration with domestic and international groups and agencies, implements capacity and training needs assessment addressing the social welfare workforce, volunteers, and psychosocial care providers in sub-Saharan Africa, and serves as technical advisor in a USAID-funded Twinning Project with the Tanzania Social Work Associations. She staffs the National Committee on Lesbian, Gay, Bisexual, and Transgender Issues and previously staffed the International Committee and Women's Issues Committee. Ms. Tomaszewski has expertise in policy analysis and implementation addressing gender equity, violence prevention, and early intervention, and the connection of trauma and risk for HIV/AIDS and other sexually transmitted infections. She has more than two decades of social work experience as a counselor, advocate, educator, and program administrator. Ms. Tomaszewski is a member of the IOM Forum on Global Violence Prevention. She holds a B.S.W. and an M.S.W.

from West Virginia University, and a graduate certificate in procurement and contracts management and a certificate in leadership development from the University of Virginia.

Robert J. Ursano, M.D., is professor of psychiatry and neuroscience and chair of the department of psychiatry at the Uniformed Services University of the Health Sciences and founding director of the Center for the Study of Traumatic Stress. He is widely published in the areas of posttraumatic stress disorder and public health planning for the psychological effects of terrorism, bioterrorism, traumatic events, and disasters, including war. Dr. Ursano has more than 300 publications, is the co-author or editor of 8 books and is editor of *Psychiatry: Interpersonal and Biological Processes* and senior editor of the first *Textbook of Disaster Psychiatry* (Cambridge University Press), which was published in 2007. He was the first chair of the American Psychiatric Association's Committee on Psychiatric Dimensions of Disaster. Dr. Ursano chaired the development of the first APA's Treatment Guidelines for Post-traumatic Stress Disorder and Acute Stress Disorder. He has received the DoD Humanitarian Service Award and the highest award of the International Traumatic Stress Society, the Lifetime Achievement Award, for "outstanding and fundamental contributions to understanding traumatic stress." He is the recipient of the William C. Porter Award from the Association of Military Surgeons of the United States.

Jeffrey Victoroff, M.D., conducts two areas of research: behavioral neurology and political psychology. With regard to the first career, he studies the neurobehavioral bases of human aggression and behavioral complications of traumatic brain injury. He has published in multiple peer-reviewed journals, is a member of the Research Committee of the American Neuropsychiatric Association, and is a program director of the National Football League's Neurologic Care Program. With regard to the second career, Dr. Victoroff studies individual factors and evolutionary imperatives that may predispose to violent extremism. He serves on the UN Roster of Terrorism Experts and has edited two books on this subject: *Tangled Roots: Social and Psychological Factors in the Genesis of Terrorism* (2006) and, with Arie Kruglanski, *Psychology of Terrorism: Classic and Contemporary Insights* (2009). His latest work for the U.S. Government's Strategic Multilayer Assessment Program was titled *Applied Evolutionary Neurobehavior to Reduce Participation in al-Qa'ida in the Arabian Peninsula*. Dr. Victoroff received his B.A. magna cum laude in great books from St. John's College, his master's degree in social science from the University of Chicago, and his M.D. with honors from Case Western Reserve University School of Medicine. He completed his residency in psychiatry at Harvard's McLean Hospital and his residency in neurology at the Harvard Longwood Medical

Area neurology program. He completed his fellowship in neurobehavior at the University of California, Los Angeles. Since then he has been a member of the faculty of the University of Southern California Keck School of Medicine, where he now serves as associate professor of clinical neurology and psychiatry. He is board-certified both in neurology and in psychiatry, and certified by the United Council for Neurologic Subspecialties in behavioral neurology and neuropsychiatry.

Charlotte Watts, Ph.D. (*Planning Committee Member*), is a professor in social and mathematical epidemiology and founding director of the Gender Violence and Health Centre (GVHC) at the London School of Hygiene and Tropical Medicine (LSHTM). An internationally renowned expert on Violence Against Women, and on Gender and HIV, she has more than 15 years of experience in HIV and violence research. Originally trained as a mathematician, with further training in epidemiology and public health, Dr. Watts brings a unique, multidisciplinary perspective to the complex challenge of addressing women's vulnerability to violence and to HIV, with a strong commitment to drawing upon the multidisciplinary expertise of GVHC to conduct rigorous, action-oriented research to inform change. Dr. Watts has held several senior research and advisory positions, including acting as a core research team member for the WHO Multi-Country Study on Women's Health and Domestic Violence; chair of the Expert Working Group to Assess the Global Burden of Inter-personal Violence; advisor to the UK Prevalence Study of the Mistreatment and Abuse of Older People; and chair of the Public Health Benefits Working Group of the Rockefeller Foundation Microbicide Initiative. She has served on several WHO Expert Consultations on HIV, on violence against women, and on microbicides, and was Track C co-chair of the Microbicides 2006 conference. She regularly gives presentations at national and international meetings, and at LSHTM teaches Ph.D. and M.Sc. students.

Deanna L. Wilkinson, Ph.D., M.A., is currently associate professor in the Department of Human Development and Family Science in the College of Education and Human Ecology at The Ohio State University, where she conducts research and teaches on urban youth violence, community processes, and violence prevention. Her research explores the causes and consequences of adolescent aggression, how it varies across and depends on contexts, and how it might be prevented. Most broadly, her work examines the ways in which community institutions and processes, as well as more microlevel and sometimes ephemeral dynamics, shape violent behavior. Her long-term goal is to clarify how structural, cultural, and situational factors intersect to produce violence and America's responses to this violence. She is also very interested in translating research for policy and practice so that knowledge necessary for solving complex problems actually transfers. She is the 2008 recipient of the Society for Research on Adolescence Young Investigator Award. She was honored at the 13th annual Strategies Against Violence Everywhere (SAVE) awards in 2009 with the Les Wright Youth Advocacy Award. In 2010, she received the College of Education and Human Ecology's Dean's Distinguished Service Award for her devotion to community service in Columbus. She received the 2010 Fire and Focus Award as well. In 2011, she was honored as "Woman of the Year" by the I'm Every Woman National Expo. Professor Wilkinson earned her Ph.D. from the School of Criminal Justice at Rutgers University, her M.A. in criminal justice from the University of Illinois at Chicago, and her B.A. in sociology from Cornell College in Mt. Vernon, Iowa.

Jamil Zaki, Ph.D., is an assistant professor of psychology at Stanford University. His research focuses on the cognitive and neural bases of social behavior, and in particular on how people understand each other's emotions (empathic accuracy), why they conform to each other (social influence), and why they choose to help each other (altruism). He received his B.A. in cognitive neuroscience from Boston University, and his Ph.D. in psychology from Columbia University.